GROWING OLDER, STAYING YOUNG

ALICE FAYE

WITH DICK KLEINER

GROWING OLDER, STAYING YOUNG

DUTTON 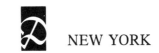 NEW YORK

DUTTON
Published by the Penguin Group
Penguin Books USA Inc.,
375 Hudson Street, New York, New York, U.S.A. 10014
Penguin Books Ltd,
27 Wrights Lane, London W8 5TZ, England
Penguin Books Australia Ltd,
Ringwood, Victoria, Australia
Penguin Books Canada,
2801 John Street, Markham, Ontario, Canada L3R 1B4
Penguin Books (N.Z.) Ltd.,
182-190 Wairau Road, Auckland 10, New Zealand

Penguin Books Ltd, Registered Offices:
Harmondsworth, Middlesex, England

First published by Dutton,
an imprint of Penguin Books USA Inc.
Published simultaneously in Canada
by Fitzhenry & Whiteside Limited.

First printing, April 1990

1 3 5 7 9 10 8 6 4 2

Library of Congress Cataloging-in-Publication Data

Faye, Alice, 1915–
Growing older, staying young/Alice Faye with Dick Kleiner. —
1st ed.
p. cm.
ISBN 0-525-24856-0
1. Aged—Health and hygiene. 2. Aged—Medical care. 3. Beauty,
Personal. I. Kleiner, Richard. II. Title.
RA777.6.F38 1990
613'.0438—dc20   89-38844
                                                            CIP

Printed in the United States of America

DESIGNED BY EARL TIDWELL

Unless otherwise noted, all photographs courtesy of Alice Faye

Grateful acknowledgement is given for permission to quote lyrics
from "Some Little Bug Is Going To Find You" by Benjamin Hapgood Burt,
Roy Atwell, and Selvio Hein. Copyright 1915 Warner Bros. Inc.
Copyright renewed. International copyright secured. All rights reserved.

I am eighty-five years old, and thanks to the Pfizer Five contained in this book I am enjoying the same activities I did forty years ago. Please believe me. It works.

PHIL HARRIS
September 1989

GROWING OLDER, STAYING YOUNG

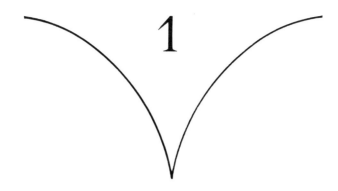

1

In the course of my life I have been paid many compliments. I imagine this is true of anyone who has had any sort of career in show business: Being complimented goes with the territory. We get a lot of brickbats tossed at us, too. If we have any smarts, we learn to ignore both the compliments and the brickbats, because both are usually insincere.

Still, it is always nice to be complimented. Some of the compliments that have come my way are marvelous. I will always treasure the fact that Irving Berlin, perhaps our finest composer of popular songs, once said, "I'd rather have Alice Faye introduce my songs than anyone else." Darryl Zanuck, when he was running my studio, 20th Century–Fox, told a reporter, "No one can sell a song quite as well as Alice Faye." And I am proud of the compliment the American moviegoers paid me when I was named the top box office star of 1940.

Through the years many other compliments have been paid to me by critics and fans and people in the motion picture business. But I think the one that has meant the most to me was one I heard not very long ago. I was attending a meeting of young elders (I much prefer this terminology to "senior citizens" or "people in their golden years" or "old folks") and I overheard one lady say to another, "That can't be the Alice Faye I used to see in the movies—why, she would be ancient, and this one still looks great."

"Looks great," of course, is a relative term. If beauty is in the eye of the beholder, then "looking great" is in the mind of the observer. But I believe I can be reasonably objective about myself—people in show business have to have a certain objectivity because, after all, how we look is a tool of our trade—and I think I can safely say that I don't look half bad for a dame of seventy-five.

Actually, in terms of my figure, I have proof that I haven't changed that much. My weight is still virtually the same as when I was in my prime—and I always think the phrase "in one's prime" makes one sound like a side of beef. When I was doing all those love scenes with Tyrone Power and Don Ameche and John Payne, I weighed around 120, give or take a pound or two.

I still do. I don't think I have varied more than 5 to 7 pounds in all those years. I've been up to 125, which I can handle pretty well. And I've been down to 115, which is a touch too light; my face looks drawn when I weigh that little. And that drawn quality in a face tends to become exaggerated, somehow, with the advancing years. So I try to stay around 120, which seems to be the ideal weight for my body. And my scales tell me that I am managing to stick to that goal reasonably well.

Obviously, my face is not as smooth as it once was. Equally obviously, my hair is not as blond as it once was. But, considering myself as objectively as I can, I am reasonably happy with the overall picture. I am also happy with something that is probably more important than how I look—how I feel. I feel young inside, and that's the important thing. A few minor aches and pains—we all have them—but nothing major, nothing serious.

That's what this book is all about. Growing Older but Staying Young is a worthy goal, I believe. Why shouldn't all of us, men and women alike, try to look and feel as young as we possibly can? Not for our egos—although there is nothing wrong with having an ego and catering to its whims—but for our health and well-being. After all, a youthful appearance and a youthful attitude toward life are signs of a healthy mind and a healthy body. If we look, feel, and act youthful, we stand a better chance of living longer. And enjoying those extra years.

How, then, do we go about cultivating the goal of Growing Older but Staying Young?

Let me say right now that I am not an expert at anything. I am certainly not a doctor or a scientist of any kind. I am not an exercise guru or a nutritionist or a makeup wizard. All I am is a seventy-five-year-old lady with a pretty decent face and figure. The only credentials I have are that I have lived quite awhile and survived without any deep scars. So all I can do is to tell you what I do to keep my face and figure looking decent. I will tell you a few things I have managed to learn in those seventy-five busy years. They have worked for me, and that's about all I can say. No promises, no guarantees, no nothing.

To begin with, I have learned that luck has a lot to do with how you look: the luck of the draw; the luck of the genes you happen to have been born with. You had nothing to say about it. If your parents and grandparents were fat and died in their fifties, chances are you will be fat and odds are you will die in your fifties, too. Unless, of course, you do something to counteract what's in your genes.

I lucked out. My parents and my grandparents were on the slim side. My Grandmother Moffitt lived with us when I was a girl. She was Irish—born in Dublin—and a feisty lady. She lived into her eighties. Back then, eighty was a very ripe old age indeed. She died when I was twelve, and she was the one who encouraged me the most to go for my dream—show business. My mother worked hard all her life, and she lived well into her seventies, too.

So I think I started out in life with a few genetic breaks. But there is, of course, considerably more to how we look and how long we live than those inherited characteristics. They may give you a head start, a fine framework for your life, but it is up to you to add flesh to that framework.

I believe I got another break when I chose my career. I started out by dancing—singing and acting followed in due course. And dancers, by the very nature of their work, are forced to exercise. Back in those days—the Dark Ages, as my rotten grandchildren love to tease me by saying—nobody exercised just for the sake of exercising. Physical fitness was unheard of. People walked only out of necessity, not for the good it might do their bodies. I don't think the terms "jogging" or "pumping iron" had even been invented yet. So chances are I would not have exercised a single muscle if it had not been that I was required to by my profession. But I did dance, so I was forced to exercise.

It wasn't until much later in my life—when I was around forty or so—that I gave any serious, conscious thought to the state of my body or the condition of my health. You will read more about how that happened later in this book.

Anyhow, the luck of my genes and my career gave me a headstart toward Growing Older but Staying Young. But even if you don't have these blessings—if your family's genes seem to indicate trouble ahead and your career forces you into a sedentary life—you still can age beautifully. You have to work a little harder to achieve Growing Older but Staying Young, but it is very possible.

My natural fair coloring was a help to me, too. Because I am a blonde (not quite as blond as I appeared in my early films, but still a blonde), the coming of some gray into my hair was not the traumatic experience it is to some brunettes. I was able to make the transition from blond to gray haired without any major shock to my nervous system.

That is why today, when people compliment me about the fact that I don't look *seventy-five,* it doesn't turn my head. I know that a lot of it is nothing I can take personal credit for. Still, it is undeniably pleasant to hear such things. After all, I may soon be a great-grandmother. I have a married grandson, so a great-grandchild is a very definite possibility. Incidentally, I wasn't able to attend my grandson's wedding, which was a big disappointment to me, and I am sure to him, too. I was working—off on a tour somewhere in my job as spokesperson for Pfizer Pharmaceuticals. I guess it is typical of modern living that my grandson probably explained my absence by saying, "No, my grandmother couldn't make my wedding—she was working."

I have always worked. And most women I have known have worked, too. To me, it is the normal thing.

In my days as a Hollywood star, I worked hard. So did all the other women—from the stars to the wardrobe ladies and hairstylists and extras. People who only view Hollywood from the outside, I have learned, have the wrong idea about what goes on on a movie set. It is no country club.

Actually, I think it has gotten more difficult in recent years. In my era most films were shot in the studio, so there were certain creature comforts available—such as air-conditioning and the proximity of bathrooms—that are not present on location. And nowadays virtually all films are shot on location, to give them admirable realism.

My last film, *State Fair,* was one of those shot on location. It was very difficult. We were in Texas, and it was hot. We were outside most of the time, and, of course, we all were supposed to look fresh and beautiful, but in those 100-degree-plus temperatures, looking fresh and beautiful is difficult. So it was a grueling and uncomfortable few weeks for me. But it was part of the job.

Remember, making a movie is business. And a very peculiar business. If I didn't show up for work, the work stopped. It wasn't like a department store, where if one clerk stayed home with an ingrown toenail the store still opened. If Alice Faye stayed home during the shooting of a film starring Alice Faye, the whole thing shut down.

And a movie is a million-dollar production, or more. Every day when no film is shot costs the production company thousands of dollars. Maybe hundreds of thousands of dollars. All the other salaries must continue to be paid. The camera crew is paid, and stands around. The electricians are paid, and stand around. Likewise the propmen and the carpenters and the makeup people and the script supervisors and the director—the whole gang is there, waiting, being paid.

I was part of some major, big money productions and, of course, part of some small money productions as well. In the darkest depths of the dreadful Depression, I starred in *George White's 1935 Scandals.* I do not know what the budget was for that film, but I do know that money was a consistent problem. Not only did they cut corners, but they often cut the whole enchilada. I remember the producer coming to me once and asking me to take it easy on the bottled water—"It costs seventy-five cents a bottle," he reminded me—so, being the cooperative young lady I was, I curbed my thirst for the balance of the shooting.

On the other hand, I was in *Alexander's Ragtime Band* in '38, and by then the recovery had set in and money was no object—or as near to being no object as it can be with Hollywood moguls. The budget for that film I remember, because at the time it was astronomical—$2 million. And the film took two years to finish.

One set was adorned with seven crystal chandeliers, which had been imported from Czechoslovakia. Each one weighed a ton and a half, all beautifully polished crystals, and they were gorgeous. I hinted around about getting one of them—of course, I had no place to hang it—but the hint was not taken. I often wondered whatever happened to those chandeliers.

So I went to work every day, no matter how lousy I might have felt. That's one of those things people don't think of when they consider the "glamorous" life of a movie star. With the entire responsibility of a huge production on your shoulders, you jolly well go to work every day.

And while you're at the studio, you do your job. With me, mostly that meant singing and dancing. You know, some days you just don't feel like singing and dancing. And, anyhow, when you have to sing the same number a dozen times or more, and rehearse your dance steps over and over until your feet are bloody lumps, singing and dancing somehow lose a lot of their joyous quality.

With it all, though, I must admit that I had a ball. Work, sure, but it was a lot of fun, too. Looking back from the vantage point of forty or fifty years later, I think I was living a fairy tale. I was the real-life heroine of something Hans Christian Andersen might have written had he lived in the twentieth century.

Think about it: In a fairy tale the heroine lives in a castle, well protected and continually looked after, and there is a procession of handsome princes seeking her hand. Well, under the old Hollywood system that existed when I was a star, the studio (20th Century–Fox in my case) was my castle. Even though we kiddingly referred to it as "Penitentiary Fox" because of its strictness, it was a refuge. It protected me and looked after me. And who could ask for more handsome princes than my leading men, gentlemen such as Tyrone Power, Don Ameche, and John Payne?

But fairy tale though it might have been, it was tough, demanding work. In those days studio contract players—such as I was—were hustled from one film to another. Today an actor considers himself overworked if he appears in two films a year. We used to do four or five and think nothing of it. It was not unusual for me to finish one film in the morning, have lunch, and start working on another picture that same afternoon.

I liked the studio system at the time, and, in retrospect, I still believe it was good. At least it was good for me. The studios protected the stars they had under contract. For one thing, there was a continuity to one's career; they tried to advance you from small parts to bigger ones to biggest ones. For another thing, the studios carefully monitored publicity. Our names and faces and reputations weren't smeared all over those sleazy supermarket tabloids, like those of the poor stars of today.

I realize that some stars—Bette Davis and Olivia De Havilland pop quickly to mind—chafed under the studio system. They didn't like the regimentation and the total control the studio moguls had over their lives. But I couldn't help but think, If this is slavery, I'm all for it.

Of course, Bette and Olivia and the rest of the rebels were girls with ultrastrong egos and ultrapowerful personalities. My own ego was practically nonexistent. I used to look at some of my fellow actors, and I would envy the bursting egos I'd see. There I would be, unsure and unsteady, wondering why I was there and how I could possibly justify the big money I was getting and the luxurious life I was leading. And I'd read stories about Alice Faye in the papers—stories the studio publicity department had planted—and I would wonder who that girl was. It didn't sound like anybody I knew.

It wasn't that I disliked myself, or felt that I should be deported to some desert island or Siberia. I just didn't think I was anything special. I didn't think I would ever stop any traffic with the way I looked or the talent I possessed. I was all right, but certainly nothing sensational. That was my honest assessment of myself.

And yet, there I was, starring in big movies opposite big male heartthrobs, getting the gigantic buildup in all the newspapers and fan magazines (which were very important at that time) and on radio (no TV then, of course). And I was beginning to make some impressive money. It all made me feel I was something of a fraud. It was an uncomfortable feeling.

In my later years I learned—the hard way—to stick up for my rights, stand up and assert myself. Nobody is going to push me around anymore—not even myself. But I was pushed around a lot in the old days, simply because I wasn't sure enough of myself to speak out. My feeling then was that I was a star under false pretenses, so whatever anybody did to me I had coming.

At the time, however, I wasn't given to self-analysis. I just did what they told me to do, and the only thing I really knew or cared about was that I was enjoying my life. I may not have felt that I deserved all the luxurious living that was being thrust upon me, but I was smart enough to take it and thank God for it.

It was, truly, a beautiful life. I did have the good sense to recognize that and to appreciate and enjoy it to its fullest. I was living the life of a paper doll. My mother—she had come out to Hollywood with me from the East—and I lived in an apartment building owned by Mae West for a time. (I visited her once, and her apartment was just what you'd expect Mae West to live in, a white-and-gold place. Even the piano was white and gold, and the carpets were ankle deep, and it all reeked of a heady perfume.) Later, when my brothers came out to join us, I rented a beautiful home and we had our own swimming pool. I haven't been without my own pool ever since.

I was recently interviewed by a young reporter who asked me what the difference was between the Hollywood of my era and the Hollywood of today. "What's missing in Hollywood today?" she asked me.

"Love is missing," I said. "And caring is missing." When you made a film back then, it was done with love and with care. It seems to me today's moviemakers don't give a real damn if you have a light on your face or not; all they want to do is get the shot in the can before five o'clock, so they can tell the accountants—the accountants and lawyers really control the industry nowadays—that they are still on schedule and on budget.

I can remember when they would spend an hour or more making sure the lighting was perfect. Fortunately, I didn't have to stand there while the electricians adjusted and readjusted the lights and the reflectors. That's what stand-ins were for. My poor stand-in would have to be on the set for that hour or more while they played around with the lights and shadows. I would be able to stay in my dressing room in comfort, reading or talking to somebody or resting. Often, however, I would have to use that time to rehearse a dance number or a song.

When I was a Hollywood star, we shot each scene from many angles and perspectives. There were long shots and over-the-shoulder shots, medium shots and close-ups and dolly shots—all kinds of shots. Today they have one camera, and they strap it onto the cameraman's shoulder. Then they shoot a scene once, and that's it. It's all done quickly and cheaply, with about as much loving and caring as you'll find in your neighborhood cockfight pit—and that's the way it looks, too.

What I didn't know then, and didn't realize until very recently, was that all that loving and caring was actually preparing me physically and aesthetically for my young-elder years.

Hollywood has always been accused of creating and perpetuating the cult of youth. The stars were all young and beautiful. Nobody ever seemed to grow old in Hollywood. We had some older character actors—people such as C. Aubrey Smith and Jane Darwell—but they probably were born old. Who could ever imagine a young C. Aubrey Smith, or Jane Darwell in pigtails? And, similarly, who could ever imagine an elderly Jean Harlow or a doddering Robert Taylor?

I was a big part of that cult of youth, innocently. I was always young in my films—even when I played Lillian Russell, they never showed her in her later years, only in her prime. In *Alexander's Ragtime Band* the script followed the two leading characters—me and Tyrone Power—for a quarter of a century, but neither of us aged a bit through it all. So I had the idea pounded into my head that it is important to look and feel young.

That cult-of-youth concept may have been a bad thing to foist on the American moviegoing public, but it subconsciously helped me to my present state. Everything I did then was geared toward looking and feeling young. Although I was unaware of it at the time, I was doing all the right things. I exercised regularly, via my dancing. The studio was constantly checking on my weight—the camera cruelly magnifies every extra pound—so they carefully watched what I ate. (I got so tired of cottage cheese and broiled lamb chops that to this day, I don't particularly enjoy eating either of those things.) And, of course, the rigors of the shooting schedule required that I go to bed early and get a good night's sleep, so I did very little late night carousing.

That was true of most of the stars. The gossip columns would be full of news about this couple being seen in that nightclub, dancing until dawn. Most of it was completely untrue—when we were working, we didn't dare stay up late. I would have to get up at four in the morning, to report to the makeup people and the hairdressing people and the costume people at the studio in time to be ready to start shooting when the working day began. Who's going to stay up until three if she has to get up at four? Most of the stuff that was printed about me and the others was invented by the studio publicity men and women.

So I was leading a healthy life, even though I wasn't conscious that that was what I was doing. I just did it because it was my job. I happened to be lucky, in that my job had all those built-in healthy aspects.

Of course, it could have been even healthier. There was no gym, for one thing. On today's movie lots and in today's television studios, there is usually a gym where the people can work out before or after shooting, or during their breaks. When Mary Tyler Moore had her show, she would personally conduct dance classes during the lunch hour. But in my era that sort of thing was unheard of. Gyms were for broken-down prizefighters, that's all. No lady would ever be caught in a gym; today going to a gym is a very fashionable thing for ladies to do. They even pump iron. The closest thing we had to a gym was the dance studio, where we would practice our routines and rehearse our numbers. I spent many grueling hours in the Fox dance studio.

I had plenty of company there, and elsewhere on the lot. We were like a family. It is, I realize, somewhat corny and almost a cliché to say that, but it was true. The old studio system was an extended family, truly—from the patriarch (Louis B. Mayer or Adolph Zukor or Jack Warner or, in my case, Darryl Zanuck) down to the lowest grip, we were part of the studio team, part of the family. From working together so closely on so many pictures, we knew everything about one another. We knew all our foibles, our innermost secrets, our hidden dreams and hush-hush desires.

There was Tyrone Power. I had met him early in his career, and I was certain that one day he would be a big star. He was a delightful person, and I wanted to help him any way I could. So I agreed to appear with him in his screen test. And so, since I had helped him when he was only a beginner, he always felt particularly close to me. Ours was always a good friendship, never a romantic one. He would tell me about his love affairs, I would tell him about mine. It was a brother-sister kind of thing.

Ty Power was one of the most handsome men this world has ever produced, with an inner nature and spirit that were as handsome as his exterior. But he didn't have much of a head for business. He was always being taken by somebody— if it wasn't his agent, who was a conniver, it was his uncle, who was another one. I don't know what might have happened had he lived, but I have a hunch he might have had serious financial problems in his later years.

John Payne, on the other hand, was very smart with his personal finances. Jack Oakie was also very sharp, but Jack Haley was the smartest of them all in that regard. He tripled his money, but he had a lot of help from his wife, the brilliant Flo Haley.

Most of us were normal, well-adjusted people. I know folks in Podunk and South Cashewnut like to think Hollywood stars were mostly crazy and totally immoral—an orgy a night—but the truth was quite the opposite. Most of us were straight arrows and very sane, simple, possibly even dull folks. There were some exceptions, of course, but there are some kooks in South Cashewnut, too.

I never saw anybody take any drugs at any party I attended in Hollywood. Today, I imagine, that has changed, but I don't go to Hollywood parties anymore. When I did— and I went to all the big ones for a lot of years—there was drinking, naturally, but I never saw any drugs.

Of course, it was a pruder and primmer era. When I did

a film called *You Can't Have Everything,* in '37, they gave a small but interesting role to Gypsy Rose Lee. She was famous, or infamous in those bluenose days, as a stripper, and the Fox brass, led by Darryl Zanuck, were afraid that the public would be outraged if a striptease artiste was in one of their films. They had visions of a public outcry and pickets in front of theaters and all that—and it very well could have happened.

But they still thought Gypsy had talent—which she did—and wanted her for the film. They solved their dilemma by using her but billing her with her real name, Louise Hovick. So if you ever watch that movie on some late, late show, you'll see Gypsy Rose Lee, but when you see the credits, you'll see the name Louise Hovick.

We had our tragic figures. I think the most tragic was Judy Garland, a sad little girl. What started her on her decline, I believe, was the strictness of her studio—MGM—and, in particular, the rigid harshness of the studio boss, Louis B. Mayer, regarding Judy's figure. She had a tendency to put on weight. So they regulated her diet so stringently that the poor girl was practically a victim of malnutrition. Then, so she would have the vitality they wanted in front of the camera, they dosed her with uppers. And downers afterwards. It became a particularly vicious circle.

Jean Harlow was another sad one. I felt a strong empathy with Jean because, when I started at Fox, they tried to make me "another Harlow." There was always that desire, among the studios, to create "another Gable" or "another Stanwyck" or, in my case, "another Harlow." So they dyed my blond hair even blonder—made it platinum blond—and plucked my eyebrows and made me slink around movie sets. That lasted until I did *Poor Little Rich Girl* in 1936.

So I felt a bond with Jean, and when she died I was terribly upset. The truth of her death was that she had appendicitis, and her mother, who was a devout follower of Christian Science, would not allow them to operate. "You don't put a knife to my darling daughter," she commanded, and they had no choice. The result was that Jean's appendix burst, and she died of peritonitis.

Another kind of mother was Shirley Temple's. I worked with Shirley on two films—*Poor Little Rich Girl* and *Stowaway*—so I got to know the Temple family very well. Mrs. Temple was, as we say nowadays, a laid-back lady. She was quiet, motherly, charming. No stage mother, she. In fact, I often wondered how it happened that she had ever let her beloved daughter near anything as raucous as a movie set. In all probability Shirley's talent was such that nothing could have stopped her from becoming an actress.

She was, as all of us who ever saw her perform recognized, a once-in-a-lifetime child. But those of us who had the joy of working with her knew that she was even more incredible than that. She was so smart it was positively frightening. She listened to the script as it was read to her, only once, and then she knew every single word of dialogue by heart. Not just her own lines, but everybody's.

And, of course, physically she was as cute as a button. Everything about her was perfect and beautiful and adorable. She even had cute feet. I used to look at her and wonder if this exquisite creature was real or not. Working with her made me want to have children of my own. I had always had the urge to be a mother, but having Shirley Temple around really intensified that desire. I couldn't wait—but I had to wait.

We all realized that when we worked with Shirley it meant nobody in the movie theaters would be looking at us. Their eyes would automatically go to Shirley. When you work with a child, or with an animal, you might as well stay home and phone your performance in. You can't possibly top them, or even match them. Without even trying, they are going to steal the scene. But that was a small price to pay. We all got such a kick out of working with Shirley that a little scene larceny didn't matter that much.

So I enjoyed my two films with Shirley. Another of my pet costars was Don Ameche. Don and I became great friends—as with Ty Power, it was purely platonic, never anything romantic—and we remain good friends to this day. I think that I absorbed something from Don subconsciously. And it was something that has stood me in good stead in my later years.

I watched Don Ameche taking care of himself physically. In those years, as I have said, physical fitness was not the widely practiced custom it is today. But Don was the exception. Every morning, without fail, he would walk. And it wasn't just a leisurely amble around the block either. Don made a point of walking eight to ten miles every day. He would tell me about his walks and often invite me to join him. I never did; I was too busy with my dancing rehearsals.

I don't think Don walked because he was consciously aware of the health value of those walks. I think he just did it because he enjoyed it. It felt good to him. If you had told him then that he was taking care of his body, he probably would have laughed at you. He would have said, "Hell, I just go out and walk because I like to go out and walk, that's all."

I could see that something was doing Don Ameche good. He had a marvelous physique and never seemed to be tired or to have any physical illnesses or problems. I believe that might have put the notion in my subconscious mind that there is some correlation between exercise and physical well-being.

I am very happy that of late Don has made a marvelous comeback in films. He is every bit as fine a character actor as he was a romantic hero. Actually, I think he was always vastly underrated as an actor. I believe he is one of the very finest actors on the screen.

Another actor I had great pleasure working with was the deadpan comic actor Buster Keaton. We were together in 1939 in a film called *Hollywood Cavalcade,* about the silent movie era. One of the scenes had us engaged in one of Keaton's famous pie-throwing fights. I have never had so much fun in my life. I guess deep down inside every one of us lurks the urge to smack somebody in the face with a lemon meringue pie. And I was able to satisfy that urge in *Hollywood Cavalcade.* In fact, I satisfied it many times, because we had to do, if I remember correctly, fifteen takes for that scene.

Of course, what made it difficult for me, and time consuming for the company, was that I started out in the scene looking glamorous and ended looking like scat. So, of course, after each take I had to go and get reglamorized. That meant a complete change of costume, redone makeup, rewashed and reset hair, the works. Between one thing and another, it took about an hour to get ready to reshoot that scene. But that was Hollywood then; nothing would do but total perfection.

I wish I had gotten to know Buster Keaton a little better than I did. He was a quiet, reserved gentleman and not easy to know. And I was never too outgoing myself, so the result was that we were polite and friendly, but nothing beyond that. I am sure I could have learned a great deal from him, if only I had tried a little harder to draw him out of his shell.

As a normal, healthy girl, with normal, healthy desires, I was in a delicious position being a Hollywood star. Remember, I'd starred in my first film when I was eighteen, and I continued to be a star until I quit when I was thirty. And there I was, this kid from the sidewalks of New York, without any education to speak of, without any real theatrical training, hobnobbing with all the glamorous people in Hollywood. Why, every girl in the world envied me.

The truth is, I envied myself. I wished I could have shaken myself up and made myself more of an extrovert. I wished I could have been more of a party girl. But like a leopard with those damned spots, I couldn't change what I was—or what I wasn't. I was basically shy and introverted, unsure of myself and totally devoid of ego.

I was just about the least-likely-to-be-a-Hollywood-star kind of person there was. But I did manage to have some fun and games. Remember George Brent? Handsome, suave, debonair George Brent. I had an unending crush on him for some time. I never got to work with him, however, so the crush went unrequited—for a while. But then we met at a party, and—oh, happy day—he asked me out for dinner. I was as excited by that date as any girl, any age, anywhere. You can make the girl a Hollywood star, but underneath she's still just a girl.

He turned out to be a charming escort, as many other girls in Hollywood had discovered. Bette Davis had a big thing for him, too, and so did Ann Sheridan. He married Ann, but that didn't last too long. When his career was over, he moved to Ireland—he had been born in Ireland and told me he always longed to go back—and spent his last years there, breeding horses and leading the quiet country life.

I had other brief sparks of romance, like any girl would in that situation. But this book isn't about my life, it is about the way I live now. And, as for all of us, much of how I live today has its roots in the kind of childhood I had.

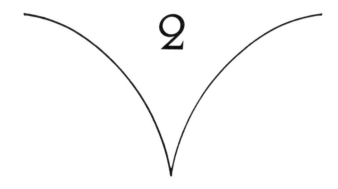

2

I may, as I have said, be a
great-grandmother. I never knew my own great-grandparents. In fact, I only knew one of my grandparents. That was
my mother's mother, the remarkable lady who lived with us
when I was a girl.

That was in New York. It was that part of the West Side
called Hell's Kitchen, which always sounds as though it must
have been an awful place to live. But in reality it wasn't bad
at all. Actually, it was reasonably pleasant.

My father was a policeman. My mother worked, too—for
a perfume company and for a candy company. I get a kick
out of today's crop of militant feminists who talk about "liberated women" as though this were a brand-new concept.
When I was a kid growing up in New York, almost all the
women were liberated. It was either that or take in washing.

I didn't know any better, so I thought I had a pretty good life. It wasn't until many years later that I ever heard that phrase "a deprived child" and realized they were talking about kids like me. I guess I was deprived, if you measure deprivation in terms of worldly goods, because we had very little. But what we did have was a warm, loving family—my parents, my grandmother, and my brothers, Charley and Bill.

Charley would take me to Central Park when it snowed and pull me around on the sled. I have a picture somewhere of my big brother pulling me on that sled of his, with me sitting there like some princess, my little muffin hat perched on top of my head. I also fondly remember going to the maypole dancing in the park. And when New York sizzled in those July or August dog days, we would sit on the fire escapes and wait until somebody turned on the fire hydrants, then scamper down and dash through the rushing, cold water.

And there was school, and church—we were Episcopalians, and we went to church, although not regularly—and all the usual things New York kids enjoy. I had my own special pleasures. I guess I was a little odd, but I loved it when somebody died—not anybody close to me, of course, but somebody whose death meant I had to attend the funeral. A funeral, you see, gave me the chance to ride in a car, which was a major event in my young life. And not just any run-of-the-road car either, but a big, beautiful, long, black car.

Hell's Kitchen was a very integrated neighborhood. There were people like us—my family name was Leppert; my father came from German stock, and my mother was Irish. And there were Jews and Italians and Poles and blacks. We politely called them Negroes then, and they liked me, I guess because I was so fair, with my hair so blond it was almost white when I was little. I remember I'd go home with one of my black girl friends and her family would call me Snowball.

My childhood was normal as far as my health was concerned. The usual childhood diseases, but nothing particularly dire or threatening. I remember equating warm feet with well-being; if my feet were warm, all was right with the world. If, on the other hand, my feet were cold, I was very uncomfortable. If my mom really liked me that day, she'd give me a hot water bottle when I went to bed and I would curl my feet around its delicious warmth. Bliss!

If I caught a cold, the official family remedy—I guess this was from the Irish side of my family—was a hot toddy. Butter and sugar and whiskey and rock candy and lemon, all warmed up and served steaming and bubbling in a big mug. I thought that was very nifty. My tummy got warm and, with the hot water bottle comforting my feet and the hot toddy comforting my tummy, I was in Heaven. I think I even looked forward to catching a cold, just so I could get the cure.

So it was a pleasant childhood, there on the streets of New York. But I guess subconsciously I knew there must be more to life. I was always dreaming of something better, something grander.

I would sit on the fire escape—my favorite place to dream—and fantasize. One of my favorite fantasies was a country one. I would think how wonderful it would be to come from a little town in the country somewhere, and I could visualize it so clearly in my imagination—the pretty house with the big lawn and the big trees, and a lake close by where I could fish. The trees were all fruit trees, and I would usually have an apple in my hand in that fantasy, or sometimes a peach, freshly picked from my very own tree.

Another fantasy involved my future husband. I knew he had to be a person of elegance. I was very impressed, at the time, by tuxedos—to me, they were as elegant as you could get—and so my fantasy was that my husband would be wearing a tuxedo. I mentioned that to my mother one day. "Ma," I said, "when I grow up I am going to marry a man who wears a tuxedo."

"Waiters wear tuxedos," she said dryly, and that effectively ended that fantasy.

I also would sit on that fire escape and dream myself into a world where I was a movie star. I loved the movies, although there was no particular star I idolized. (Later, after I became a star myself, I came to idolize Bette Davis and Joan Crawford, because I knew how hard a job it is to be a good actress on film, and they were both so marvelous.)

It is really rather incredible how many movie stars did come out of that New York environment—James Cagney and Ruby Keeler were both from a similar neighborhood, for example. I imagine that they, too, sat on fire escapes and dreamed those big dreams. I know I did, and my dear grandmother encouraged me to go out and try to do something about making those dreams become a reality.

My first job, when I was twelve, was working at a dancing school. I worked in the dressing rooms, and about all I remember of that job was that I had to take care of the tap shoes. But I remember very distinctly watching the lessons, and picking up some tap dancing steps along the way. I would watch the pupils doing their thing, and then I would go home and do it myself.

That was the extent of the lessons I had—until I got to Hollywood, where the studio system then was really one vast graduate school for performers. But I never had a singing lesson in my life—I am still, regrettably, so ignorant about the technical aspects of music that I don't even know what key I sing in—and the only dancing lessons I had were when I snooped during those few months I worked at the dancing school. But I guess I had some natural ability, because I picked up those tap steps very easily. And I sang naturally, too.

I was also growing into a woman. When I was thirteen, I was already pretty well developed, and by the next year I could pass for eighteen or nineteen—and did. After grammar school, the itch to begin my show business career was so strong that I decided I had to scratch it. I began working that year, as a chorus girl.

One of the reasons I was able to pass for an older woman was that I was well endowed. To some girls that is a source of pride, but to me it was always a source of embarrassment. Later, when Betty Grable and I did our famous "Sheik of Araby" number in the movie *Tin Pan Alley*—it had boys and men all over the world drooling—we had to wear very revealing outfits. I was so busty and so embarrassed about it that I wore a shawl over my costume until the last possible second.

Betty, on the other hand, was just the opposite. Her figure had to be given an assist; the costume department supplied what Mother Nature had neglected to. She envied me, Betty said, and I know that I envied her. And we laughed about it. She could wear dresses I never could, and vice versa. So we never borrowed each other's clothes. (By the way, all that stuff about a feud between us was just something the Fox studio publicity department dreamed up to draw attention to our films. The truth was that we liked each other very much and became good friends, and stayed good friends until the day she died.)

But the point is that I was then so terribly embarrassed about the fullness of my figure that I begged the Fox executives to let me wear costumes that would hide God's (and nature's) generosity. But, of course, Darryl Zanuck and the rest of the 20th Century–Fox brass tried to show as much of me as the standards of those days would permit.

Thus I did pictures such as *Lillian Russell,* and Lillian was a lady who was known for her bustiness. And that "Sheik of Araby" number from *Tin Pan Alley.* And others like it. I wasn't exactly the Dolly Parton of my day, but I wasn't Twiggy either. In fact, I was very distressed when, in its review of my second film, *Now I'll Tell, Variety* used only one adjective to describe me: "buxom." They could at least have said "blond" or "beautiful," but all they said was "buxom Alice Faye."

Of course, by today's standards what we did wouldn't even be considered slightly naughty. Not a single eyebrow would be raised. With the amount of nudity there is on the screen today, absolutely not a thing is left to the imagination. In my era, even though they might have pushed the illusion of bare skin, the reality was something far different. I remember on many occasions being sent back to the dressing room by a studio censor because my gown was cut too low. And a few times we actually had to reshoot entire scenes that did not meet the exacting standards of the Hays Office, which supervised movie morals in those days.

I think they went too far in one direction—primness and bluenose prudence—but many of the films of today go overboard in the other direction. There is, or should be, a happy medium. I hope someday we will find that happy medium in our motion pictures.

Of course, when I look back at the way I felt during the filming of that "Sheik of Araby" number, I have to laugh at myself. What was I so damned uptight about? But that was the way I was, then. Mostly, I think it was because I was so unsure of myself. I had no self-confidence and very little sense of pride in my own worth. Oh, I was well aware of the fact that I had done something very few people my age had done—become a motion picture star when I was still a teenager—but I couldn't help but wonder, Why me?

I would try to assess myself, take stock of my assets, and, in truth, I didn't think I was so hot. Not too bad to look at, but I was certainly not one of the greatest beauties the world had ever known. My figure? OK—except that I was convinced I was too busty. Voice? OK, too—I could sing pleasantly, but Lily Pons was not quaking in her booties. Dance? Again, all right—but Fred Astaire would never point a finger at me and say, "I want you!"

One thing I did have going for me, even though I was only eighteen when I became a movie star, was experience. I had begun when I was only thirteen. At that time I had auditioned for, and been hired by, the Chester Hale dance units. I started with them at the Capitol Theatre, in New York. It was hard work, right from the beginning. I may have had some notion about show business being glamorous, but if I did, that notion was quickly knocked out of my head. We girls worked too hard to have any time for glamour.

The show at the Capitol changed every week. So while you did the existing show—four or five times a day—you were also rehearsing for the next week's show in between performances. I was actually getting a lot of very healthy exercise. Silly me, I just thought I was being worked like a dog. If I had only known, I would have paid them for letting me have all those terrific aerobic workouts. Sure I would.

So, by the sheerest accident, I was leading a very healthy life. I don't remember too much about what I was eating in those days—probably not very much—but when you're doing a tour of one-night stands, or doing a couple of shows a day in the chorus line, you eat when and where you can. We hoofers ate mostly at greasy spoons, and I guess I ate a lot of unhealthy fried stuff. But when you're young, your stomach can take a great deal of abuse. These days I eat well, and I have no problems in that department.

It was my connection with Rudy Vallee (I was the vocalist with his orchestra) that brought me to Hollywood. He was then the big radio singing idol—a heartthrob such as Crosby and Sinatra and Presley and Springsteen would become—so naturally Hollywood summoned him. He was put in a film called *George White's Scandals,* and Lilian Harvey was set to be his leading lady. They said I might have a small number somewhere. But Lilian Harvey, an English-born beauty, was more of a dramatic actress, a Garbo type. And this film was to be light, a bit of froth. She was wrong for the part, and she knew it, and soon the studio knew it, too. Rudy suggested me for the part, and they tested me, and they said, "OK, it's yours."

At the time the story was circulated and printed all over that Lilian Harvey had demanded her role be expanded and quit when they refused. That, so the story went, was how come I was given the part. But the truth was that she was simply not right for the role as it had been written.

I had lied about my age from the beginning. I was actually born in 1915, but I said I was three years older, so many of the reference books still list the year of my birth as 1912. But in 1933, the year *George White's Scandals* was made, I was actually only eighteen. I don't believe there has been another girl who starred in a major movie as a teenager, except perhaps Sue Lyon in *Lolita,* and that really doesn't count.

I danced in almost all my films, and when we danced in pictures, we danced! We rehearsed and rehearsed and then we rehearsed some more. So I had no choice. I exercised, and I stayed slim and trim and fit, although still I never thought of it as exercise or fitness training. I just called it work, with a lot of fun mixed in. I really thoroughly enjoyed my years as a movie star. A lot has been written about the studio system, and a great many actors and actresses did chafe under its rigidity; some openly rebelled. It was rigid, there is no question about that. The studio regulated your life, down to the most minute detail. You had no choice of the parts you would play; they were all assigned to you, and you played them or else you were suspended without pay. The studio told you what lessons to take, how to do your hair and your makeup, what clothes to wear. They selected the people you would date for important functions. They told you how much money you would make, and, unless you fought them, they would bank it for you and only let you have an allowance. They told you where they wanted you to live.

It might have been considered a trap, but if it was, it was that well-known one made of the richest velvet. If it was a cocoon, it was lined in satin. If it was a prison, it was the most luxurious prison ever conceived by mortal man. I sometimes felt the urge to break out, to make a few decisions of my own. But more often I just leaned back and relaxed and enjoyed it all.

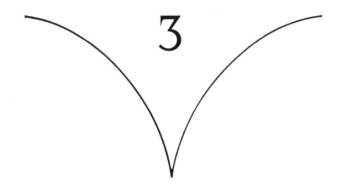

3

One of the things that made my life, when I was a Hollywood star, so enjoyable, was the people I met.

Outsiders reading about Hollywood have developed, I think, an entirely wrong picture of the old movie stars. They think of them as self-centered, spoiled, temperamental, childish. Undoubtedly some of them were—but I'm sure you will find plenty of self-centered, spoiled, temperamental, and childish folks among your circle of acquaintances, too. My point is that Hollywood stars are like any other group of people—you'll find some good folks and some bad folks in any crowd.

Most Hollywood stars were good people. When my mother and I first reached California, we rented an apartment in Hollywood itself. George Raft lived in the same building. If you remember him, he was the typical tough guy, at least on screen. But to us he seemed to be simply a very sweet and generous gentleman. He took pity on us, two green-as-grass newcomers. And he loaned us his car and chauffeur. So until we got our bearings we toured the city courtesy of that tough guy George Raft.

I had never learned to drive and, of course, neither had my mother. As a matter of fact, I was very much afraid of automobiles. That fear dates from my days with Rudy Vallee and his orchestra. As we toured I was in two bad accidents with Rudy, which left scars on my body and my psyche, too.

Once, after finishing an engagement in Atlantic City, we were in a big Cadillac touring car. We were en route to our next stop, which was Virginia Beach. Rudy was driving, I was sitting next to him, and there were three members of the band in the backseat. Rudy apparently fell asleep at the wheel, and the car went off the shoulder and flipped completely over. My lower back took the brunt of the fall, and I have had lower back problems ever since that day.

Another time Rudy and I and his car wound up in a ditch in Maine. That one wasn't so bad, but still it was scary, and I've been nervous in and around cars ever since.

I drive myself, of course. But I won't do any long drives, and I won't drive in the dark. I guess I am a sissy, but anybody who has been in a serious accident will understand my paranoia. I drive to the market and back. Period.

One question people always ask me about Phil, my husband, concerns his drinking. In his days with Jack Benny, he was famous because he supposedly drank a lot. Today, when I am such a strong advocate of good health—and excessive drinking obviously is not a very healthy thing to do—it is only natural that people would want to know how I reconcile the two.

While Phil might have toasted a friend now and then, he was never an excessive drinker. That guzzling of his was pretty much a gimmick, a way to get laughs—like Benny's supposed tightness with a dime, which also was greatly exaggerated. Phil is justifiably proud of the fact that, even though he drank his share, he never failed to do his job, and to do it very well. He never missed a show or a cue in his life. But Bing Crosby, his very good buddy, used to say that if Phil was ever going to write a book, he should call it *To My Liver, with Love*.

Phil and Bing stayed healthy by walking a lot. Phil still does. He is a tireless walker, tramping all over the desert with his black Labrador retriever at his side. Phil and Bing used to go to Mexico very often, down on the Baja, and walk the mountains, shooting quail and jackrabbits.

Bing would call Phil "The Indian," and the name caught on with the Mexicans. Phil did look a lot like an Indian, with his face burned a dark copper by the sun, his habitual red kerchief tied around his head, his gun slung across his shoulder. All that walking has obviously helped him. He's eighty-five now, and still in great shape. A few aches and pains, but he looks a lot younger than eighty-five, and feels a lot younger, too.

"If I'd known I was going to live this long," Phil always says, "I'd have taken better care of myself." (It's an old joke, but who knows? Phil may have said it first. He's an old jokester, after all.)

And I believe I look considerably younger than my seventy-five years, too. I know I feel much younger, very much younger. Most of the time, that is. There are moments—we all have them—when time catches up with us. But if you are careful, you can avoid most of those moments.

A few years ago, as an example, I was traveling for Pfizer, and at some airport I had to change planes. The connection was tight—I had only a few minutes to make my next flight—so I ran across the airport to reach the gate on time.

Big mistake.

In running, somehow I hurt that sensitive lower back area, the one that has given me problems since that time the car rolled over when I was driving with Rudy Vallee. Because of aggravating that problem, I was unable to do my usual exercising for a month or so. I must tell you, I was a very unhappy woman during that time. I could literally feel my body changing, because I couldn't swim and I couldn't walk and I couldn't do any of the things I do—which I will tell you about in detail in later chapters—that keep me in shape. And these things also keep me happy, because I am convinced there is a direct correlation between your physical condition and your state of mind.

Deterioration was setting in because of that enforced idleness. It was just a little over a month, but it happens that fast. All the good I had been doing all my life was being wiped out in the space of not much more than thirty days.

I made myself a promise then. Never again would I be so foolish as to run across an airport to catch a plane. It just isn't worth it. There will always be another plane, but I have only one back. And I'm not about to trade my back to catch some damn airplane. That isn't an even swap.

So since then I have become a little more careful in what I do and what I don't do. I don't run in airports. I don't try to tote a lot of hand luggage myself (skycaps have to live, too, so I let them do the toting and I tip them and save myself a few aches and pains). In fact, I simply do not overdo anymore. I figure that is a small sacrifice to pay in honor of my seventy-five years. It doesn't mean that I am limiting my activities, merely that I am being prudent.

I have to do a lot of traveling in connection with my work for Pfizer. I'm sure I travel much more than the average person. Since I did so much traveling when I was younger, on the road as a performer, I do not particularly enjoy traveling anymore. It is, however, a necessary evil if one wants to go from Place A to Place B. So I travel. These days it is almost always by plane, and I must confess that I am not the world's most cheerful flyer. If the truth be told, I am not too happy up there. As soon as I step aboard a plane, I can feel myself tense up. The moment I disembark is a very pleasant one.

I remember very fondly the old days of train travel. I made that cross-country trip so often—the Chief from Los Angeles to Chicago and the 20th Century from Chicago to New York. It was, in those days, a great way to travel. You relaxed. The food and the service were both superb. There was no tensing up when I got on board the train.

But time and travel arrangements march on. So today, like it or not, I do a great deal of flying. It does have its good side, of course, which is the time factor. I can visit so many more places and thus meet so many more people when I fly. And I am enjoying meeting all the wonderful people who have written to me over the years. I find it amazing—and very heartwarming—to realize how loyal my fans have been.

And it has been a long, long time for them to have remained so loyal. After all, I started in pictures in 1934, with *George White's Scandals,* and my last film was *Fallen Angel,* in 1945. (Film students will say, "Aha! I caught you! You forgot *State Fair.* It's true, I did come out of retirement in 1962 to do *State Fair,* mostly at Phil's urging, but that was a bad mistake—and a bad picture, notable only for being the vehicle that introduced Ann-Margret to movies.)

So, with that one unfortunate exception, my fans have been loyal for more than forty years without seeing me up there on the screen. I did do radio, of course, for many years, and I made many television appearances in those four decades, but movie fans are movie fans and don't really count the other stuff. Yet these wonderful fans of mine have stuck with me and kept writing to me, and now, when I travel for Pfizer, they are there to say hello to me by the hundreds in whatever city I visit.

They have been with me through thick and thin. I have

led, I believe, a fortunate life, and there has been more thick than thin. But I have had my share of disappointments and body blows.

My first marriage, to Tony Martin, didn't work. We had met when he had an unbilled bit in a film I did called *Poor Little Rich Girl,* and the romance flourished and the public was very excited about it. We did *Sally, Irene and Mary* together just after we were married, and our fans were so anxious to see us together that they made that so-so film a major box office smash. But the marriage simply did not work out.

I married Phil, on May 12, 1941, even though a lot of my good friends advised me against it. They said it would never last. In fact, I have been told that a lot of Hollywood plungers were actually betting real money on just how long Phil Harris and Alice Faye would stay husband and wife. Well, that was more than forty-nine years ago. We are closing in on our golden wedding anniversary, and we are still hanging in there.

Maybe one reason is that we were married twice. Not many people know this, but we were first married in Mexico—we thought that sounded romantic—but I wasn't sure it was legal, so, when we came back across the border to Galveston, Texas, we got married again, just so it was good and binding. That wedding in Mexico, since it was impromptu, was a wild affair. Nobody had remembered the bride's bouquet, so one of our friends ran across the street to a vegetable patch and picked a head of cauliflower and a couple of carrots and some lettuce leaves and made a bouquet out of all that.

Years later, when my daughter Phyllis was married, she had an elegant bouquet designed by a very fashionable florist, and the basis of that arrangement was a head of cabbage, with flowers intertwined among the leaves. It made me think back to my own cauliflower-carrot-lettuce bouquet, and I felt maybe it was good luck to carry something old, something new, something borrowed, and a couple of vegetables.

It hasn't always been easy. No marriage ever is. There simply have to be some moments of doubt, of panic, of conflict, along the way. You have to ride them out, as a sailor rides out a storm at sea. I believe that one reason so many marriages today break up after only a few months or a few years is that nobody seems to be willing to bend even a little. If some problem comes along, some dispute or disagreement—and such things are inevitable—the only answer today's young people seem to have is to walk out, to break up. That is their only solution to a dispute. Just go see a lawyer and get a divorce, or, if they aren't married, just pack up and move out.

It never would occur to them to compromise, to give a little here and there. And if a marriage is to work, you must learn how to compromise. You must be able to make some concessions, to have some flexibility, to bend before you break. Phil and I have had our problems, but we both feel our marriage is worth saving, so we have saved it. It has often taken some hard work, but we have done it.

One of our own secret weapons for a successful marriage has always been to give each other some privacy. Or, as they say these days, some "space." We don't believe that a marriage means that both parties to it must be forever joined at the hip. He does his thing—going off to golf tournaments, zipping down to New Orleans to sit in with his musician pals Pete Fountain and Al Hirt, going hunting or fishing—and I do mine. We are together a lot, but we are apart a lot, too.

When two people—any two people, no matter how compatible, no matter how much they may love each other—are together all the time, there is bound to be some friction. They get on each other's nerves. Allowing the other some time by himself, by herself—some "space"—is one way to lessen that friction and avoid a lot of useless, unnecessary bickering.

And I am convinced that bad moods—the kind that useless, unnecessary bickering brings on—can affect your health and physical well-being. Scientists have proven that there is a correlation between your mental and physical states. I do not claim to understand the physiological happenings in the body, but I know what happens to me. If I sink into a bad mood, in a very short time I don't feel well. A headache, or indigestion, or just a generally blah feeling. I can make myself a nervous wreck in nothing flat, and all because of a bad mood.

So I try to avoid them, and one way Phil and I do that is to cut down the chances of our irritating each other. If we are apart from time to time, then the times we are together are less likely to produce those frictions, that unpleasantness, those bad moods. It's good for us as people, and it's also good for our health. And the healthier I feel, the younger I feel. It is that simple.

I used to have a temper. Not a terrible one, but still I could blow my top occasionally. It happened most often when I was at work. I would get annoyed at inefficiency, and I would yell a little. But I have learned to control it. When you lose your cool, that can also bring on some physical problems.

And we all have enough physical problems without manufacturing new ones when we throw a temper tantrum. As far as I am concerned, the most important thing in the world is to feel good, physically and mentally. Whatever little upsets happen—and they are bound to happen—can be dealt with if you feel OK.

So I wake up every morning and check all my moving parts to see if I'm still here and still functioning. Most of the time I feel wonderful in the morning. I thank God that everything is in operating condition. Another good day. That's the way I look at it. That's the way I start every morning, or try to, by feeling fine and thanking the good Lord for that feeling.

I believe that one reason I feel good 99 percent of the time is that I made the correct choice when I decided to quit making movies after *Fallen Angel* in 1945. Very few Hollywood stars have walked away from the fame, the fortune, and the hullabaloo. I was only thirty at the time, and I had plenty of scripts being submitted to me. So it wasn't that my career was finished or that I was over the hill or that nobody wanted me anymore. There was plenty of life left in the old girl.

It was simply that I was tired of it all. As I have mentioned before, I never had much of an ego, nor did I have a great deal of ambition. When I went into pictures, back when I was really not much more than a child, at eighteen, it was fun and exciting—and a very pleasant way of making a living, which was something I had to do. But then Phil and I were married and we had had two children—Alice Jr. was born on May 19, 1942, and Phyllis on April 26, 1944—and the need to earn a living was no longer hanging over my head. Phil made enough for all of us.

I might have stayed and done a few more pictures, if I could have done the kind I wanted to do. After all those years of light and flimsy musicals—pleasant enough and good entertainment, but hardly anything you could call meaty—I longed to sink my teeth into a script that had some bite to it. It is, I suppose, the old story of the comic who yearns to play Shakespeare. Or at least George Bernard Shaw. I didn't exactly want to play Shakespeare or even Shaw, but I knew I could handle something more dramatic than dancing to "The Sheik of Araby." So I asked Darryl Zanuck to let me have a dramatic role in my next film.

"No, Alice," he said. He was polite and he was smiling, but there was a patronizing air about him. "No, my dear, I see you in another lovely musical. After all, that's the Alice Faye the public wants to see, isn't it? A little singing, a little dancing, a little romancing. We have to give the public what it wants, don't we? That's our business, after all. So run along now, like a good girl, and keep on practicing your dance steps."

And that was that. So I walked out. End of one career.

But the end of something is always the beginning of something else. So the end for Alice Faye, movie star, marked the beginning for Alice Harris, housewife and mother. I segued from one career to another without missing a beat. Phil and I had a home in Encino, in the San Fernando Valley, at the time. And I threw myself into the unfamiliar waters of housewifery. It was sink or swim, because I really knew nothing about this new job.

I had never done anything around a house. As a kid in New York, I helped my mother around the apartment, of course, but life on the West Side of Manhattan is a lot different from life in an affluent Los Angeles suburb. I had done a little basic cooking, but not even very much of that. And that was the extent of what I knew about running a house. I had never even marketed. When I was a child, my mother had sent me to the corner grocery store to get things, but that was just a question of giving the man my list and lugging the bag home. Then later, when I had my own home, there was always a housekeeper to take care of the shopping, as well as most of the other details of running the house.

At that time I still hadn't mastered the art of driving a car. No need. The studio had always sent a limo to pick me up, take me to work, and bring me home again in the evening. I had never diapered or bathed a baby. I had been too busy working, so we had had a nurse to do all that sort of thing. Now I was home, and I had to do the shopping and the cooking and take care of two babies, both under three years old.

So I was dumped, willy-nilly, into those unfamiliar waters, and I spluttered and I struggled, but I survived. I learned how to do everything by trial and error—mostly error, but I learned and Phil was patient and the babies didn't know any better, so they were patient with me, too.

I learned the hard way. Take doing the marketing. The first time I went to the supermarket, I did it all wrong. I didn't know how to buy things. So I came home with cases of soap and one potato. I thought one potato equaled enough mashed potatoes for the whole family. I had cases of some stuff and very little of other things. It was all backwards.

Phil took a look at what I had brought home and laughed. "What is all this stuff, honey?" He shook his head in amazement. I don't think he knew whether to laugh or cry. "Look, baby, you don't buy a case of jars of olives. You buy one jar at a time. But you really should buy more than six grapes. Next time, buy a whole bunch of grapes."

Phil knew more about running a household than I did at first. Back home in Indiana, his mother had taught him a great deal about working in and around a kitchen. In fact, he is a fine cook—his corn bread is a thing of beauty. But I have learned, through the years and through experimentation, and now I am no slouch around the stove either.

Still, until the day I quit being a star, I really had not learned how to live. I know that may be hard for people to believe—the predominate picture is that movie stars really live it up, and maybe some of them do. But not little old me. I had led a quiet, almost a sheltered life. I may have known how to sing and dance and act, and I could decorate a party nicely, but I knew nothing about the important things—running a house, raising children, coping with a husband.

So for the next ten years or so, I didn't do much else but conquer that new field of endeavor. I did work with Phil on our radio show, but that was a ball—easy compared with movies or television. The radio show was a snap, and it satisfied what little urge I had to do any performing.

All my old Hollywood friends had told me I would miss the action around the studio. "You'll be back," they had all said. "You'll find yourself going stir-crazy, stuck in the house all day long."

But that never happened. I found I didn't miss anything about being a movie star. Oh, perhaps there were a few twinges when I thought about the fun we'd had on the set, the joking and the laughs and the camaraderie. But that was more than offset by the joys of being a mother, of watching Alice and Phyllis change every day before my eyes, of being a witness to that miracle of nature that is a growing child.

So I was content. In fact, like most women, I believe those years when my daughters were young and totally dependent on me were the happiest, most fulfilling years of my entire life.

There was one cloud on my otherwise blissful horizon. But that cloud would ultimately prove to be one of my greatest sources of pleasure. One day I woke up to the realization that I wasn't paying any attention to myself, to me, to Alice. I had become so wrapped up in all the many facets of my new housewife career that I had forgotten that I owed some allegiance to Alice Faye.

I hadn't exactly gone to pot. As I wrote earlier, my weight has never varied much, so I hadn't grown fat or sloppy. But I simply did not feel as alive and energetic as I once had. I was tired a lot of the time—I had a right to be tired, of course, because being a housewife is a physically demanding job, but I felt I was more tired than I should have been. I would collapse into bed not long after I had put my daughters to bed, and had done the dishes, and had taken care of Phil's clothes, and all the rest of it.

I would fall into bed about nine, without even enough energy left to do any reading or watch any television. And that wasn't like me. I had always been full of energy. I could do a day's work and then dance the night away, and never drop a stitch.

It came to me one day that I was suffering from the same

problem athletes have when their careers are over. A football or baseball or basketball player, when old age catches up to him and he has to retire, generally has a very difficult time adjusting to idleness. And that is why so many ex–professional athletes die young; their bodies cannot accommodate the new life-style. The smart ones, I had read, continue with some form of exercise so their bodies can make that adjustment. And this is true for female athletes, too.

I realized I was in danger of going that route. After all, I had been as physical as any athlete. I had used my body as much as any football player. Maybe there hadn't been any physical contact, but my muscles had worked just as hard. So I would have to learn to adjust, too, if I wanted to stay fit for the rest of my life.

Just about that time, by a happy coincidence, I received an invitation to go to the Elizabeth Arden salon for a complimentary analysis and workout. I went, and that was the beginning of the new me. I went through a session at Arden's, and I came home feeling great. I realized immediately that my body demanded that I keep active. It was used to activity. I had been dancing since I was very young, and it was essential, if I was to stay healthy and fit, that I continue. So I did.

That very day I began a program of physical activity. Actually, it dignifies my exercise routine to call it a "program." That implies a rigid schedule, and there is nothing rigid about the way I keep physically active.

It seems to me that many men and women are frightened away from fitness because of that very thing, because they are afraid of being regimented, afraid they won't be able to stick to any regular schedule. They don't want to have to be told to go somewhere, two or three times a week, at a certain hour, for their exercise. They don't want to have to be told to do sixteen deep knee bends and then chin themselves sixteen times. I don't blame them. That kind of thing would turn me off very quickly, too. There is nothing worse than being forced to hew to a set, rigid schedule. It takes the fun out of anything.

So let me tell you right here and now that the program I advocate isn't really a program at all. It is all very informal. You do what you want to do when you want to do it. If you don't feel like doing anything today, don't do anything today. I always remember that great quotation from the immortal baseball pitcher Satchel Paige: "Whenever I feel the urge to exercise, I lie down until the feeling goes away." Of course, if you follow his advice every day, you'll never get any exercise at all. But you can be like Satchel Paige a couple of days a week and enjoy yourself and still stay in shape.

What I do is walk when I feel like walking, swim when I feel like swimming, do some stretching exercises when the urge comes over me to do stretching exercises. And I feel wonderful.

I believe I average a strenuous workout of one kind or another three or four days a week. I am very fortunate in having my own swimming pool, and swimming is one of the great pleasures of my life. So I will jump into the pool almost every day, but some days I just swim around idly for fifteen or twenty minutes or so. On other days, when I feel the need for something more strenuous, I do some serious swimming and some special exercises (which I will tell you about in Chapter 7); I really give my body a genuine work-out on those days.

Of course, Growing Older but Staying Young isn't only a question of staying physically fit. There is a lot more to it than that. Your mental attitude is also an important part of the formula.

After I had found that I needed exercise for the physical side of my continued well-being, I next began to tackle the mental side. That did not have quite as clear-cut a solution.

But again, I believe I was fortunate because of the career I had chosen for myself so many years before. Whereas so many people—men and women alike—fear the onset of the years, people in the acting profession often welcome it. That's because the really great acting parts are usually written for mature actors and actresses. When you are young, and categorized as an ingenue if you are a girl, or a juvenile if you are a boy, the parts are generally pretty dull and routine. But as you get older and your face begins to mature, you become qualified to play the more interesting roles.

I remember when I worked with Ann-Margret in *State Fair.* She was a gorgeous thing, but she had a driving ambition to prove that she was a good actress—eventually she did prove it. She told me she couldn't wait until she became old enough so they would let her sink her teeth into a really dramatic role, not the silly young thing she was playing in *State Fair.*

Look at my old pal Don Ameche. People laughed at the parts he played when he was young. He laughed at them, too. He did a remarkable job, I always thought, in making the most of those dull parts. Now that he's in his eighties, however, he is happily being cast in much more challenging roles.

So actors, if they have any drive and ambition, do not fear the coming of their older years. Of course, there are some movie and TV people who fight it, because their only assets are their youth and good looks, but they are not real actors, they are just personalities, so we will forget about them.

I think I had become imbued with the actors' idea about the older years being nothing to dread. Still, when I hit my fortieth birthday, and then my fiftieth, I had to stop and reassess my life. When my daughters grew up and got married and became mothers themselves, I had to reexamine who I was and where I was going.

I came to some conclusions after that reassessment. To stay young, I believe, is a three-pronged proposition.

First, there is your health. Now, obviously, as we get

older there are more and more things that can go wrong with us. Many of those things are beyond our control. But most of them are in areas over which we do have control in varying degrees. And even the things we cannot control can often be eased these days. I will get into all of that later.

Next, there is physical fitness. This is related to health, but it is not quite the same thing. Health is the absence of disease. Physical fitness is having a body that is in excellent working order—a heart that is pumping efficiently, lungs that are clean and clear, a circulatory system that functions well, and muscles and joints that move smoothly and painlessly.

Finally, there is your mind and your general state of mental health. You can't look or feel young if you are not happy, and you can't be happy if your mind is in a state of disarray. You have to create a mood of peace and tranquillity in which to function. The best way to do that is to stay active. Boredom breeds mental unhappiness.

I believe wholeheartedly in that statement, and the facts bear me out. We have all heard of some relative or family friend, active and healthy all his life, who reaches retirement. Then, within a few months, he passes away. Without something to keep his mind occupied, he became so unhappy that he couldn't face life and his body rebelled, so he died.

Part of a healthy mental state is appearance. The better you look, the better you feel. More on this later, too.

Health, physical fitness, mental health—those are the three prerequisites for Growing Older but Staying Young. I will talk about all of them in detail in subsequent chapters.

As far as my own life is concerned, I have had a few problems with my health. Nobody can totally avoid them. I have a bit of arthritis in my hands, and I have high blood pressure, but this is controllable these days and mine is under control. I have already told you how I discovered the need to keep physically fit when I was forty. As for my mental fitness, I have always been active, and I still am. I could never just vegetate. That's not me. So when people compliment me these days on how I look, I am pleased. But I know that we can all look, feel, and act younger than our years.

Here's how.

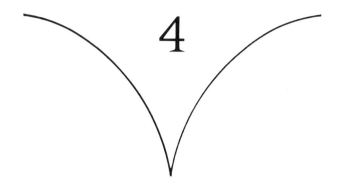

4

I think we Americans are blessed with the ability to find humor in almost anything. Even getting older. I remember hearing that wonderful comedienne Moms Mabley, near the end of her long and remarkable career. She was talking about old age, and she said it isn't a very hard thing to attain. "One morning, you wake up, and you got it," she said.

And Bob Orben, one of the best and certainly one of the most prolific gag writers around, once wrote about getting older: "I don't need birthdays to remind me that I'm getting older. My body does it for me."

My own favorite line about aging may strike some as funny, but it is really a very serious thought. And it happens to be very true. That is, I don't worry about getting older—I worry about *not* getting older.

Just look at the obituary page in your local newspaper any day. Men and women in their forties and fifties are dropping like flies. And it is certainly not uncommon to read about some poor soul dropping dead of a heart attack at thirty-six or so. These days, with the tension of modern living and the pace we must maintain just to keep up with the pack, it is surprising actually that more of us don't fall victims to an early death. So that's why I say I worry more about *not* growing old.

Scientific studies have shown that the leading causes of death are directly related to the way we live. There is, they say, a very definite link between how we live and whether we will survive to reach our young-elder years. There are other factors that contribute, of course—such as heredity and luck—but the way we live is the paramount cause of death and disability.

If we smoke heavily, for example, our chances of living to a ripe old age are vastly diminished. If our job is full of stress and tension, ditto. If we eat a diet full of fats and salt and sugar, likewise. If we let ourselves become obese, the same thing.

All those ways of living—and scientists call them "risk factors"—increase the likelihood of early death or early heart attack or early stroke. But it should be very obvious to you that all those risk factors are surface things and can be changed. You have total control over your life-style. You can stop smoking, stop eating unhealthy foods, stop putting on so much extra weight. So you do have a certain amount of control over how long you are going to live.

I was in Atlantic City, New Jersey, not too long ago, and I went for a long walk on the boardwalk one morning. I couldn't help but notice how terribly out-of-shape most people are. There they were, fat and sloppy, walking along with great big ice cream cones in their faces, or munching on hot dogs, or carrying bags of saltwater taffy and chewing away.

A lot of them were so fat they had difficulty walking. And they were young, too, which made it even sadder. They were snacking their lives away. There were some older ones, which was bad enough, but the younger ones were an even sadder spectacle.

I couldn't help but remember an old joke. Maybe Phil told it to me; as I have said, Phil is the world's biggest repository of old jokes. Anyway, this one is in the form of a question.

Q: What's the greatest contraceptive for people over fifty?
A: Nudity.

In most cases it is all too true. And the saddest thing is that it is so unnecessary. With a little bit of self-restraint and a little bit of thought and care, people can look great and look sexy well past fifty. Life—and beauty—is not the sole property of the young.

But those people on the boardwalk in Atlantic City were obviously unaware of that. There they were, oblivious to the beauty of nature around them—the waves crashing on the sand, the gulls circling above, the glorious clouds in the blue sky—and stuffing their faces with French fries and Popsicles. All around them was beauty, and they were creating ugliness, letting themselves go to Hell.

We are in control of our lives, to an extent that is great and getting greater all the time. We are in a position to make positive changes in the way we live. And these changes can, in return, have a positive effect on how long we live and the quality of those future years.

My doctor friends tell me that in the new branch of medicine called geriatrics—the study of the problems and diseases of old age—they have reached the conclusion that the main enemy is not the process of aging itself but the diseases that can afflict the elderly.

Every year progress is being made in conquering these diseases, or at least mitigating their effects. So every year the possibility of living longer becomes greater. In Japan today the life expectancy has already reached 80 for women and 74.5 for men. A figure of 100 and even 120 is well within reach.

The Japanese have a longer life expectancy than we do. And, incidentally, the Japanese in Japan have a longer life expectancy than the Japanese in the United States. Similarly, the Italians in Italy outlive the Italians in the United States, and the Norwegians in Norway outlive the Norwegians in the United States, and so on with almost every nationality.

Why is that? They say the answer is obvious: Our lifestyle is not as healthy as it is in other countries. We eat too high on the hog—and on the cow, too. We live too well for our own good. The more we live it up, the faster we go down.

But growing old does not have to mean growing worse. We used to think that as you age, you will necessarily go downhill. You will automatically and inevitably lose your capability, your memory will go, you'll lose your eyesight or your hearing or both, you will start to dodder. Today's researchers believe this is not necessarily necessary. It is possible to grow old gracefully.

Take that legend that old folks must lose their memory. In fact, the prevailing picture of an elderly man was the absentminded professor, who would forget his hands if they weren't permanently attached to his wrists. They used to bandy around the word "senile" for anybody over sixty-five. They used to talk about a "second childhood," because of that picture of older people doing childish, forgetful things. In his book *The Mind* (New York: Bantam, 1988), Dr. Richard M. Restak writes, "The mind is not preordained to suffer an eclipse in function as we age. Indeed, it can continue to operate at its best well into the eighth and ninth decade."

"Senility" and "second childhood" are symptoms of disease—the awful Alzheimer's disease primarily, but there are others of the same sort and danger. These are truly dreadful and tragic conditions, but they really affect only a very, very small percentage of the elderly. And science is making progress in combating these diseases, too, as it is making progress in coming to terms with most diseases that affect the elderly. For most of us, growing older does not mean growing senile. The majority of people today face the prospect of later years that can, and should, be happy and fulfilling ones, without any diminution of their capabilities.

A recent study by the National Center for Health Statistics is proof. They asked people over sixty-five if they had problems in the home, with things like housework or shopping, using the telephone or preparing meals. The largest percentage of people with problems were women who said they had difficulty doing heavy housework, such as using the vacuum cleaner. Slightly more than 30 percent reported trouble in that area. But that was the biggest percentage in the entire survey. And, of course, it means that 70 percent of those women did *not* have trouble handling heavy housework. In all other areas the respondents said they had no trouble at all. So age does not have to be a time of lessening activities or heightening difficulty.

As I mentioned earlier, in my trade—acting—old age brings better parts. Of course, girls whose only talent was looking beautiful did have a problem as soon as the first wrinkles blossomed around their eyes. I remember seeing so many of the "pretty young things" begin to panic, and hysteria set in. They knew there was a busload of younger, prettier girls arriving in Hollywood every day from Texas and South Dakota. So if they showed any signs of aging, they were finished.

When I was at the peak of my career, I remember the prevailing philosophy in Hollywood was that anybody thirty-five was old. Forty was positively ancient. Fortunately, this notion has changed totally. Our whole national attitude toward age has changed, and continues to change, as more and more people become older and older. Even Hollywood's attitude has changed.

I remember once seeing a headline in the *Los Angeles Times*, something like ELDERLY MAN KILLED BY HIT-RUN DRIVER. When I read the story, I saw that the man was sixty-three. I was furious and actually wrote a letter to the editor of the *Times*, suggesting that sixty-three should hardly be considered elderly. He answered me, saying he agreed. He said that headline had been written by someone in his early twenties, "and to a boy in his twenties, sixty-three seems to be a very old age." He said the paper's policy was not to call anyone elderly unless he or she was more than eighty years old.

Nowadays, as our age span increases, we can do more and more things later and later in life. Just look, for example, at how many women today are having babies in their forties. Britt Ekland, who is well past forty, had a baby not long ago. Good for her, and good for all those women who are becoming mothers after forty. Why not? If your doctor says you can, go for it.

As long as you are healthy, age should not interfere in any way with your activities. Actually, with more and more leisure time, young elders should be able to do anything.

I know I still hope to learn to play the piano. It is one of those things I have always wanted to do, and just never got around to doing. But there is absolutely nothing stopping me from learning to play the piano, except my own laziness. I have the time, I have the interest, I have the physical capability. I don't have a piano, but maybe Phil will buy me one—although I doubt it. And one of these days I am going to sit down at some piano and accompany myself while I sing one of my old numbers. That is one of my better-quality dreams. But it is a dream that is well within the realm of possibility, as are most dreams we have as we grow older.

If we have our health, there is really very little that is

impossible. But if we don't have our health, almost anything seems to be beyond our reach.

I remember one evening when I was in New York, I was invited to join a group of people for dinner. We met at my hotel—the Sherry-Netherland—and walked the few blocks to the famous 21, where we were to have dinner. As we walked I happened to be next to a man I knew to be one of the richest men in the world. He had made billions in the shipbuilding business. And I started talking about what I thought I might have for dinner.

"That sounds good," he said. "I wish I could eat like that. But I've had problems with my stomach lately. I'm afraid I won't be able to eat much of anything tonight."

I watched him that night at 21. While everybody else was having steak or grilled salmon or veal chops, that poor guy ate milk toast. I thought to myself, If that's what being one of the richest people in the world means, you can have it. The man could have had anything he wanted—he could have bought and sold all of us at the table, and he probably could have bought the restaurant with his petty cash fund—and he had to eat milk toast.

I suppose he got those stomach problems from worrying about keeping all that money. From the superwealthy people I've known, I realize that their big worry—one that keeps them up at night and gives them those ulcers—is that people will try to take away their money.

That's not living. At least not to me it isn't. I'd rather have my health and eat what I want to eat and sleep peacefully at night than have all that money. Of course, I never want to be poor either, but enough is enough.

Peace of mind is so important to your health. That wealthy shipbuilder had all the money in the world, but it hadn't bought him peace of mind, so his health suffered.

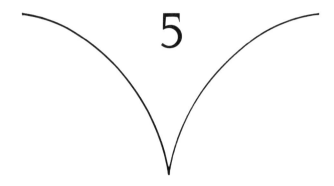

5

The first place to find peace of mind should be at home, but that is often the last place it exists.

It is hard for any two people to lead a peaceful existence. I know there are times when Phil gets on my nerves, and I am sure the vice is versa frequently, too. Phil is a very nervous man, always "on the jump," as he would say. That's why we value our privacy. I know some people don't approve, but I believe strongly that apartness is just as important in a happy marriage as togetherness. I don't believe we are put on this earth to cling to somebody else. We come in alone and we go out alone, so it stands to reason we should spend a lot of the time in between alone, too.

I believe we all—and particularly women—must learn to take care of ourselves. That's another reason why it is so important to spend some time alone. You can't learn self-sufficiency if you're always hanging on to somebody else.

And the sad truth is that the majority of women are going to become widows. Statistically, that is the hard, cold fact. I have seen so many women whose husbands have died who had been so dependent on their husbands that they are quite literally lost. They don't even know how to get gas for their car. The men have done everything for them, and without their husbands these women are poor, frightened, bewildered, lost souls.

I prefer independence for myself. I want to be able to do things for myself. Maybe that is a reaction to all those years when the studio overprotected me. I don't want anybody else doing it now. So Phil has his life and I have mine. We have many moments when we are together, when we cheerfully and happily share our thoughts and our activities, but we also have plenty of time to ourselves.

I do have time in my life for animals, however. I am a great believer in loving animals. Having dogs, especially, is a vital part of my existence. I simply do not understand people who don't love animals. I probably wouldn't like those people very much.

I've always had dogs ever since I had my own place. Right now I have a couple of marvelous poodles. I would have twenty dogs if I could. They are wonderful company and great fun. Even back when I was on the road, touring with shows, I always had a dog with me. He stayed in my dressing room or in my hotel room.

I've heard so many young elders say they are lonely. I tell them, Get a dog, get a cat, get a canary. Anything that is living and breathing, that will be company for you. You can talk to your pet—the neighbors may think you are a bit dotty, talking to a parakeet or whatever, but let them. It's your life, and if it makes you feel less lonely talking to an animal, what does it matter what the neighbors think?

I talk to my dogs. I run with them around the pool laughing out loud. Who cares what anybody else thinks? As long as they don't throw a butterfly net over me and haul me off to the funny farm, what do I care?

I like to cut loose and enjoy myself like that. I also like to talk to myself. People might think that's a bit daft, too, but I don't care. In the car I'll be talking to myself or singing, and I'll stop at a red light and see the driver who pulls up next to me do a double take when he spots me having a nice conversation with myself. So I'll smile at him and wave, and he will laugh and smile and wave back. I talk to myself and sing to myself and, sometimes, bawl myself out for doing something dumb.

Maybe I'm a little peculiar. Fine. I think it's good to be a little nuts. The way this world is constituted, I think you have to be a little crazy to survive. If you try to go through life being very sane and very straight, you'll *really* go off your rocker.

I try, every day, to reward myself in some way. Or to give myself a break in some way. That way, each day I think I am getting a little better, a little stronger.

It's all part of my belief—or perhaps it isn't so much a belief as a hope—that there is something better than this life waiting for us after we die. And the better we are here, the better we will be in that next life.

I am not a dedicated churchgoer. As I said before, I am an Episcopalian, and once in a while I'll go to a Catholic church because I enjoy the ceremony. But I carry my belief with me; my house is my church.

There are mysteries. Why did I get so lucky and have my marvelous, exciting career? Did I deserve that? What right do I have to be writing a book? I never even went to high school. My only accomplishments are that I can sing and dance and act a little and I have very nice penmanship. I was also pretty good in arithmetic; I could always add well. But I'm talking about important things in this book—how to stay young as you grow old is a very big subject—and it is a mystery to me how I got lucky enough to write about such a very big subject.

Mysteries. Another one is how we change, mentally, as we grow older. Have you noticed it in yourself? You gain confidence as you get more mature. When you are a teenager, or in your early twenties, you have the cockiness of youth. But this is more bravado than confidence; you are whistling in the dark. Then in your thirties, forties, and fifties, you know enough about life to be unsure of yourself. Finally, in your sixties, you begin to have the confidence of maturity. You can look at yourself in the mirror in the morning and say, "Good morning! You are a pretty good person. You have done a lot of good in your life. You have made a few people happy."

As I mentioned before, I never had much in the way of real self-confidence when I was young. Even when I was a big Hollywood star, I was unsure. I knew, logically, that I was an individual the world admired. There were Alice Faye Fan Clubs. My fan mail was enormous, and every day brought a couple of letters from men proposing marriage. (Some were pretty tempting, too; I remember a wealthy Argentinian cattle rancher said he would give me a 500,000-acre ranch and 10,000 head of cattle for a wedding present, and a Frenchman offered me a castle in the Alps, among other goodies.) Reporters wanted to interview me and producers wanted me for their films and there were continual offers to do radio appearances and to perform in theaters and stage shows.

All that should have turned my head. It turned the heads of a lot of other Hollywood people. But for some reason it had no effect on me. I was still doubtful of my own ability, and I could not believe all the fame that came my way.

When very important and very handsome men began courting me, taking me out and proposing marriage (and other types of liaisons), I couldn't believe they were serious.

I know that may sound naïve, but I swear I had no idea that I had any power over men. The letters poured in, with all these professions of love and adoration, and I thought they must be for somebody else. How could they mean me?

Today I have confidence. Now I believe I am something special. But this isn't conceit. It is the knowledge that we are all special. Every one of us is an individual, worthy of respect and love. So I am deserving of respect and love, too, and that is the self-confidence that comes with years.

Looking back on my life as a Hollywood star from the vantage point of today, I believe I was very fortunate to get out when I did. There I was, the great big Hollywood star, actually leading a pretty grungy life. It's probably hard for outsiders to understand, but all that glamour is just veneer, coating a pretty hard life. I wanted to be deserving of the fame and fortune, but I didn't think I deserved it.

It may sound like I am contradicting myself. I said before that it was a fairy-tale life and now I say it was a grungy life, and maybe you wonder how it could have been both at the same time. But it could have been, and it was. It was a fairy tale in that my every wish was granted and I seldom had to lift a finger, and all around me were handsome men and beautiful ladies. But it was also hollow, repetitious, and confining, and you really never could be your own person.

If I hadn't gotten out when I did, it would have eaten me up. I would have spent my life in a futile attempt to live up to my notoriety. I could never have done it, not in a million years.

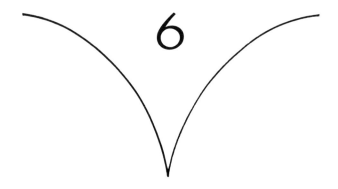

6

When I heard of the tragic and, I believe, unnecessary death of Tyrone Power, I felt, There but for the grace of God go I. Ty died in Spain, in 1958, while he was making a movie. He had a heart attack. If he had had that attack somewhere where there were modern medical facilities, chances are he would have survived. But this wasn't the major tragedy. I think the saddest thing about the death of Tyrone Power—and the thing that made me realize how fortunate I had been to get out when I did—was the heart attack itself.

Ty was the victim of the system, the Hollywood system that grinds actors and actresses down, makes them give their blood and their souls (and, in Ty's case, his life) to making movies. There is never any respite for a movie star.

I know, the public laughs when anybody says that a

movie star has a tough life. They look at the big money stars make and the gorgeous homes and swimming pools and fancy cars, and they say, "How tough can it be?" But the stars pay for all that luxury. The work is hard and the hours are long, but it is much more than that. It is the constant tension—will the picture be a bomb? Will I ever get another part? Am I losing my voice? Am I losing my hair? Do those wrinkles around my eyes show? Will the director understand what I am trying to do? Will the public accept me in this kind of part? Will my TV series be picked up for another season? Will they put a big hit opposite my show? And on and on.

Movie stardom is the most insecure profession in the world. Actors and actresses have always had to cope with rejection—there is nothing as upsetting to an unsure person as having to try out for a part—but movie stardom exaggerates this condition. Except for a very few superstars, nobody is ever sure about tomorrow in the movie star trade. All it takes is a couple of pictures in a row that fall on their faces, or a TV series or two that flop miserably, and a career can be over. Like that. Luck plays an enormous part in anyone's film career. Find yourself in a hit, and you're automatically a hit, too. Find yourself in a bomb, and you're forgotten.

In 1936 I did a movie called *King of Burlesque.* It was the first film in which my character carried the film. So when it was a success, I was a success, too. Three years later I was in a piece of liverwurst called *Barricade.* That was a genuine botch—they changed the story after we shot it, splicing bits of film together in the editing room. What finally was shown in the theaters made no sense at all. My hairstyle changed within scenes because of that haphazard editing.

Had *Barricade* been made early in my career, I might not have survived it. As it was, since I had already achieved some degree of fame and reputation, I was able to ride out the

storm and move ahead. But I have always thanked my lucky stars that I decided to get out when I did, that I got out with my sanity intact and my body whole. I have tried to keep it all clicking along that way ever since, and I think I have succeeded pretty well.

Let me share a couple of secrets with you. There are two things I do reasonably regularly, tricks that seem to make me feel good. And, as I have said, if you feel good, you've pretty well got it made.

One of the two is very inexpensive. In fact, if you happen to have somebody around the house who is the least bit handy with tools, it will cost virtually nothing. I love to lie on an angle board. Some people call it a slant board. It is simply a wooden board, slightly longer and slightly wider than an ironing board but roughly that shape. And it is placed at a forty-five-degree angle, with supports to keep it steady in that position.

I lie on that board every day for anywhere from ten to thirty minutes. My average time is probably fifteen minutes or so. And I come up fighting. I don't know what it is about that time on the board, but it does wonders for me. I just lie there, and sometimes I may doze off for a minute or so. Probably it is the angle, which makes the blood in my body flow down to my head. Whatever it is, the board seems to rejuvenate me.

I have forgotten now who introduced me to the angle board, but it was somebody back at 20th Century–Fox. The board I have now is one I got then, back at the studio. It folds up, and I used to take it on my trips, and cart it back and forth between the studio and my home.

During the war I remember reading how the medics used to treat GIs who were badly wounded by putting them on an angle board like mine. Apparently, they benefited from the blood going to their heads, too.

All I know is that, after my daily period on that board, I get up feeling like a new woman—even if the old woman wasn't so bad. I get up ready for anything.

I add to the pleasure by putting a couple of witch hazel pads over my eyes when I climb aboard. That enhances the soothing effect of the experience.

Sometimes I'll do my marketing in the morning, then come home and jump in the pool and swim for a while. Then I'll romp with my dogs for a bit. And then I'll lie on the angle board, with the witch hazel pads on my eyes, for perhaps twenty minutes.

If I know I face a long night—some dinner I must attend or a function of some kind that demands my appearance—then I will get on the board at four or four-thirty in the afternoon. That evening, which had seemed daunting just a little while before, becomes a piece of cake.

My theory is that one reason my skin and complexion are still pretty good—everyone tells me that I have the skin of a much younger woman—is the angle board. It seems logical to me that that daily dose of blood, rushing to my face as I lie on the board, cannot help but be good for the skin. That may or may not be true, but one thing definitely is true—lying on the board simply makes me feel great.

Another thing that makes me feel great is a really good massage. That is not an inexpensive item, however, and obviously not everyone can afford to hire the services of a masseuse or a masseur on a regular basis. But it is certainly beneficial, if you can swing it.

When I was just starting out, as a chorus girl in my teens, one of the biggest stars on Broadway was a lady named Mae Murray. She was famous for dancing "The Merry Widow Waltz." I remember thinking she had the most beautiful figure I had ever seen. Then I found out she was sixty years old at the time, so her extraordinary figure became even more extraordinary. I met her—the world of Broadway in those days was a small world—and I told her how beautiful I thought she was.

"What's your secret, Miss Murray?" I asked.

"How old are you, dearie?"

"I'm fifteen, but they think I'm eighteen."

She laughed. "You don't have to worry for a few years yet," she said, "but you are never too young to start. My secret is massage. I have a massage every day of my life."

I think I started getting massages when I was seventeen. Mae Murray is long gone, but I will always be grateful to her, because massages have been a joy in my life.

When I was at the studio, they had a masseuse, a great, strapping hulk of a woman who was a specialist in Swedish massage. I would get a massage from her every evening. I would come home from the studio, have dinner, get in bed, and study my lines. Then this lady would come in, give me a massage, and I'd go right to sleep. Slept like a baby, and when I got up—I'd have to get up about four to get to the studio in time for my makeup call—I would feel refreshed and ready for another long day at the office.

These days I have a massage as often as I can—usually about twice a week. Of course, the trick is finding somebody who is a good masseuse or masseur. It isn't just rubbing; there is an art (or is it a science?) to massage. If you don't have someone who is genuinely skilled and proficient, you are actually wasting your time and money. But if you do find a professional, it is a marvelous experience. And I think it is a beneficial one, too. It helps the circulation, I think, and also is great for your skin tone.

Of course, there are many people, I know, who hate the very idea of a massage. The notion of somebody doing anything as intimate as massaging their body is a total turnoff. Certainly I respect that feeling. If you don't like the idea, by all means don't do it.

All I know is that I love it. And I have read that massage

is one of the oldest forms of therapy known to man. The ancient Egyptians were great lovers of massage, as were the Greeks and Romans. So there is nothing new about it.

Recently, of course, massage has gotten a bad name because of all the publicity about massage parlors. But you can't equate a really professional massage with the sleazy goings-on in those dens.

A massage *is* a costly indulgence. There are many things that will naturally be higher on your priority list. But if you can afford a massage occasionally, by all means indulge yourself. The way I feel about it is that it makes me feel so good—and, I believe, it is so good for me—that I am willing to spend the money to get a good massage. As they say on that commercial, "I'm worth it!"

Those are two of my secrets, and you're welcome to them. Of course, you may not like either, or find either beneficial to you. We are all individuals, and we all have our likes and dislikes. As Phil says, that's what makes horse races—and it also makes the human race.

Every star I have ever known has had some private little trick that he or she likes, some special indulgence that seems to be pleasurable and helpful. My years in Hollywood roughly paralleled those of the Norwegian skating star Sonja Henie, who turned out quite a few films with figure skating as their theme. I remember her once trying to convince me to adopt the technique she used to keep her legs looking young and trim. At least three times every day, she bathed her legs in hot—really hot and steamy—water. She believed fervently that by doing this she prevented aging. We'll never know if it worked or not, because she quit Hollywood, went back to Norway, and died a reasonably young woman, in her fifties.

The point is that whatever you do, do it religiously. Nothing can possibly work unless it is done on a regular and continuing basis.

In a picture I did called *Wake Up and Live,* I sang the title song, which contained this line: "Help yourself to good health." I think that could be the theme song of this book, and also the theme song of my life.

Think about it. Help yourself to good health. That's the key. It is up to you.

There are days when I feel depressed for some reason. We all have them. Often there is no logical reason for that feeling. You just wake up and feel awful. Maybe it has something to do with the humidity or biorhythms or astrology or something. I don't know. I just know I feel way down.

When I was younger and had a day like that, I'd simply wait it out. Roll with it. I'd spend the day feeling sorry for myself, feeling lower than a snake's belly, with the only consolation being the knowledge that eventually it, too, would pass. But as I got older I came to understand I could do something about those moods. I'd wake up with that deep-in-the-dumps feeling, and I'd say to myself, "Oops, Alice, we've got one of those days on our hands. Let's get moving." So I'd do something—something "to help myself to good health," something to make me "wake up and live."

And I learned that I can work my way out of a fit of depression like that. I may simply go for a walk, briskly and brightly, swinging my arms and looking at the flowers. Or I may do some hard work, like cleaning out a closet that I've been meaning to clean out for months. Or perhaps writing some letters I've been putting off for one reason or another. The trick is to keep moving, mentally or physically or, preferably, both.

Of course, if you do not feel physically well, it is almost impossible to fight those onslaughts of depression. Without your physical health, you can't do those things—the walking or the closet cleaning or whatever—that assist you in battling your way out of the depths of gloom. So you must always try to keep yourself well. If you have that solid foundation of physical well-being, then it is possible to wake up and live, to fight your way out of the blues.

I've proved it to myself so often. There have been many times when I just felt so rotten, so low, so blah, that I couldn't face anybody or anything. But if I do a few exercises—do a few laps in the pool or something—then magically my whole mood changes. I climb out of the pool and the world has suddenly changed into a much better place and the people in it are all beautiful.

I have a hunch it all has to do with circulation. Maybe those depressed states are caused, at least partially, by some malfunction of the circulatory system. Not enough blood is reaching the right places. Then comes the exercising, and the circulatory system is forced to go to work and the blood is pumped throughout the body to all those nooks and crannies where it is supposed to be. Suddenly then everything is working and your body is happy, so your mood is happy, too. The mind must reflect the state of your body. The two are definitely related. What affects one, affects the other.

Another vital element in the overall picture of our physical and mental well-being is sleep. Scientists tell us that, as we get older, our bodies require less and less sleep. I am sure they know what they are talking about, because I realize that I can get by these days on considerably less sleep than I required when I was thirty. Still, I do like my sleep. I know some people only sleep for four hours or so and are perfectly happy, but I need more than that. I don't need the eight hours my body once demanded, but I still enjoy a good seven-hour sleep most nights.

Phil is a champion sleeper. I am usually up and about by seven in the morning, but my dear husband stays in bed longer—anywhere from a half-hour to two or three hours longer. If I'm gone on weekends, he tells me he will cheerfully spend all day Sunday in bed. I tell him that's a very bad thing—a dangerous thing. I know I don't want to get hung up in that bed. The thing is, a person can get so infatuated with lying in bed that he never wants to leave it. I'm afraid of that—afraid that if I stay in bed too long I'll never get out of it.

But a certain amount of sleep is obviously an integral part of this whole business of Growing Older but Staying Young. It's all part of maintaining your health, which is the cornerstone of aging well. Without that, nothing else really matters.

There are, of course, other factors over which we have no control—or very little control. The weather, for example. We all know how the weather influences our mood and our health. On lovely, clear, crisp days, most of us feel like we can conquer the world. On hot, humid, sticky days, we feel like we couldn't even conquer a wounded butterfly.

If we have physical problems, they are magnified by certain weather conditions. Moist days make my arthritis flare up dreadfully. But I hardly notice it when the humidity is low. Even so, I want to live in London in my next life. Maybe I won't have arthritis in my next life, so London's dampness won't bother me. But that same dampness works wonders for the complexion. I know my skin always feels marvelous when I'm in London, which is one reason I love that city so much. I feel years younger there, because my skin feels so much more youthful. I also love the custom of afternoon tea, so I'm happy as a clam in London. I hope whoever is in charge of next lives is reading this book.

To be honest about it, perhaps one reason I love England so much is that the English always loved me so much. I was extremely popular there, for whatever reason, and, human nature being what it is, we tend to reciprocate good feelings. So when the English welcomed me so warmly, I was predisposed to like their country—and I did, and I still do.

We have very little control over the climate in which we find ourselves. If we happen to be in a place where the climate is continually bad, we have the right to move. Sometimes that right cannot be exercised, however—a job or family obligations or other reasons make a move impossible. But you should seriously consider moving on if the climate is really hurtful to your health. It's something to think about.

We cannot control who we are, basically. We are born with our own set of genes, which govern so much about our lives. We can't change them. But, within limits, we can make changes in our appearances and personalities. It takes work and willpower, but we can make some alterations in those key elements.

A few changes are relatively simple—hair coloring, for example. And now, with colored contact lenses, we can even change the color of our eyes. Men can grow a beard, or take one off, to alter their appearance. The way we dress can greatly change the impression we make on the people we meet.

Other physical changes are more difficult. We cannot change how tall we are. But we can change our shape to some degree. Losing weight is the most obvious way to change, but one of the hardest for some people. Gaining weight is equally hard for some who are cursed with the problem of being too thin. But some changes can be made.

Personality changes are also possible, although with great difficulty. I know some people have been able to make profound alterations in their personalities. Introverts can force themselves out of their shells. Extroverts can sometimes learn to temper their exuberance.

But what I am more concerned with in this book are elements over which we have much more control. I think we all have it within our power to control the factors that affect Growing Older but Staying Young.

One of those factors is the amount and type of exercise we give our bodies.

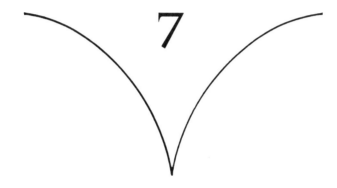

7

In this chapter, I will talk about the importance of regular exercising as part of Growing Older but Staying Young.

Let me reiterate what I said very early in this book: I am not a doctor, a scientist, or an expert of any sort. I am only going to tell you what I do, what I have learned from listening to the real experts, and what I have read. You should check with your own doctor about this and about everything before you begin any sort of regular program.

In fact, you should always check with your doctor when you embark on any major change in your life. If you read about something that somebody does—whatever it is, from a new way of exercising to a new diet—and it sounds good to you, ask your doctor if it would be OK for you to do it. Maybe there is something in your particular health picture that would make that new system of exercising or that new diet dangerous for you.

Of course, the exercise I recommend most heartily is really something that anybody can do, and that is walking. Walking has always been part of my life. Actually, I had— perhaps I still have—a distinctive walk. It was so distinctive, in fact, that critics and fans often commented about it. It wasn't the hip-swaying, seductive walk of Marilyn Monroe but more of a determined walk. In his book about my movies, *The Alice Faye Movie Book,* W. Franklyn Moshier often refers to "the Faye Walk." At one point, he writes, "She moved forth with a no-nonsense air." It was nothing I worked on or thought about. It was just the way I walked naturally, but I suppose it is all part of the body language people talk about these days. I guess my walk reflected my inner determination, so, without giving it any thought, I had acquired a way of walking that was distinctively my own.

Walking has much to recommend it. Doctors tell me that it is the ideal exercise to benefit the entire body. If you walk along at a reasonably brisk pace, your heart is forced to pump a bit harder, and every heart needs a bit of a workout from time to time. That pushes the blood throughout our bodies, meaning that our circulatory systems get a workout, too.

Swing your arms as you walk. So all your limbs—arms and legs—are being exercised.

Breathe deeply. Your lungs, too, are participating in the exercise that walking is giving you.

So virtually your whole body, head to toe, benefits from a nice, long, brisk walk.

That's the physical side of walking. I think that there is nothing as stimulating to the mind or as soothing to the spirit as a walk either. As you walk, you can let your mind wander. If you are fortunate, as I am, to live in an area of natural beauty—trees and grass and blue sky and lovely vistas—then your mind will wander easily and generally take you to serene thoughts. Even if your environment is urban, and you walk on concrete sidewalks among cars and tall buildings and have to dodge hurrying, scurrying pedestrians as you go, you can still let your mind take you to other places, other times.

What makes walking the finest of exercises, too, is one major factor: It costs nothing. Oh, you may want to invest in a pair of comfortable walking shoes, but even that isn't a necessity, as long as you have something to walk in other than your Sunday-go-to-meeting shoes.

Some people hang one of those stereo cassette players around their necks, or tuck a portable radio in their pockets and stick the earphones in their ears. If that's what you want, fine, but I personally prefer to let my mind loose to roam the world. I believe the people who carry sounds with them don't get to see the flowers or notice the birds.

I was frightened away from those stick-it-in-your-ear systems once when I had one and didn't hear the siren of an approaching ambulance. It nearly hit me; I jumped out of the way at the last possible second. So I swore off them there and then. Actually, I don't know how people can go around with their ears so busy. They actually don't know if they are coming or going when they are so concerned with what they are listening to. They often, literally, don't know where they are. To me, one of the greatest joys of walking is the freedom it allows your mind and your imagination.

I walk wherever I happen to be. I prefer my own home area, because it is familiar and safe and I love the look of the trees, the lakes, and the flowers. But I even walk when I am in New York, and the walking there is tough.

A few years ago, when I was in New York on a visit, I went shopping at Bloomingdale's. I came out, an hour later and several hundred dollars poorer, and ran across the sidewalk to catch a taxicab. I turned my foot and wound up in a cast for a couple of months. And that was just going across the sidewalk.

Still, I walk in New York. It is very hard on the feet and the ankles and the knees, but it's better than not walking at all. The problem isn't New York particularly, it is anyplace where one must walk on a concrete sidewalk or a cement street. There are, of course, many millions of people who have no choice; it is either the concrete sidewalk or staying home and doing nothing. That is all there is; it's the only game in town.

Wherever you are, as you walk you can observe nature—even in the city you can see some birds, some clouds, the sky. And, of course, in the country there is so much more to see and wonder at. I remember a quotation from the great naturalist John Muir, who once wrote, "As age comes on, one source of enjoyment after another is closed, but Nature's sources never fail. Like a generous host, she offers her brimming cups in endless variety, served in a grand hall, the sky its ceiling, the mountains its walls, decorated with glorious paintings and enlivened with bands of music ever playing." A walk in the country, to the observant walker, can be all those things.

I suggest that you keep a record of your walks—times, distance (you can estimate distance because, roughly, we walk about a mile in fifteen minutes if we walk at a reasonable clip), and other pertinent data. I am a great believer in records, not so much to tell you what you have done but as a basis of comparison for the future. If you walk a mile now in fifteen minutes, and a month from now you find you can walk two miles in twenty-five minutes, then you can quickly see how your endurance has grown, and you can set goals for yourself for future walks.

I don't want to indicate that you must always strive to go farther, faster. Actually, walking should not be a contest. We are not out to set records. In fact, I deplore those who say,

"Well, if walking a mile is good for me, then walking two miles should be twice as good." That doesn't necessarily follow. More is not always better, and twice as much is not always twice as good.

Keeping a record, however, does encourage you to walk on a regular basis. And some increases in the distance you walk and in your speed of walking those distances are valuable. As the exercise we do—walking—makes our bodies stronger, they need a bit more exercise. If we start out with flabby, unexercised bodies, we may only be able to do a certain amount of walking. But, as the flab goes away and the heart becomes stronger, we should be able to do more.

So keep those records. They do not have to be elaborate. A simple log will suffice, with the data entered perhaps like this:

DATE	TIME	DISTANCE	REMARKS
6/23/90	10:00 A.M.–10:15 A.M.	1 mi.	Huffing and puffing; Saw dog with blue overcoat.
6/25/90	10:00 A.M.–10:15 A.M.	1¼ mi.	Still puffing, but did walk a bit farther today.
6/28/90	9:30 A.M.–10:00 A.M.	2 mi.	Less huffing but still puffing. Had great idea for new invention—mint-flavored camphor balls!

You'll find it is fun to keep a log, one you can go back to from time to time, but, more important, one that enables you to see your progress. And, when those mint-flavored camphor balls make your fortune, you can look back at your walking log to check out the day the idea first came to you.

I like to walk by myself, but I know many other people prefer to have company. Perhaps they feel that in union there is strength. Maybe they wouldn't go walking if they didn't have somebody who would share the walk with them. Or possibly they are afraid to walk alone, and I can certainly understand that fear. If I didn't live in a secure area, I believe I might feel the same way.

Many people enjoy "mall walking," hiking around a shopping mall. Even if you're alone you don't feel lonely. And there are all those shop windows to look at.

However, I want to be able to walk at my own pace, stop when I feel like stopping, sing when I feel like singing, skip if I feel like skipping—without having to worry about what somebody else is doing or thinking. So I always walk alone. Once in a while Phil will go with me, but that is a very rare occasion these days.

If you do prefer company, however, go for it. In fact, you might consider joining a walking club or, if you can't find one to join, getting together with a few friends and forming a walking club of your own. There are advantages to being part of a group, like a walking club. You have an incentive to go out there as scheduled. So many of us, I know, are born procrastinators. "I'll do it tomorrow." That could be the motto of half of America. And the other half's motto: "One of these days, I must start doing some walking."

But if you are a member of a walking club that meets on a regular basis—say every Tuesday, Thursday, and Saturday morning, exactly at 8:00—then there is something pushing you to get out there and walk. And a lot of people need to be pushed. It becomes something of a social event. You walk for, say, a half hour, and then you go somewhere for brunch or coffee or maybe lunch or perhaps just to sit and chat. You get together and establish the distance you want to walk and agree on a pace you all feel comfortable with. It is a lovely way for a group of friends to spend an hour or so together a few times a week.

Walking—whether you do it alone or with another person or in a group—is probably the ideal exercise. Even if you do some other exercises, you should do some walking, too.

But don't run, don't jog. Obviously, millions of people are runners and joggers. But I find the difference between walking and running becomes crystal clear when you look at the faces of people who are walking and those of people who are running. Ever notice them? The runners' faces are contorted, strained, full of pain. Every step appears to represent a terrible effort. There is no joy there. Walkers' faces, on the other hand, are generally calm, placid, cheerful. There is no pain or strain evident there.

There are, I realize, people who subscribe to the no-pain, no-gain theory of exercise. They believe that unless your body suffers, the exercise is of no value to you. That is just so much macho hogwash. In fact, sports medicine experts have told me they advise professional athletes always to stop short of the point where pain sets in. If you have pain, they say, it is your body telling you, "Enough, already." So runners, gasping and suffering, are really doing their bodies harm, not good.

The whole point of exercise is to help your body, not to hurt it. Running and jogging can both be harmful to your health, according to the doctors I have talked to. You can put too much strain on your heart, as well as on your legs and, in particular, on your knees. To a man (or woman), they advise walking, not running, to your nearest point of good health.

As I have mentioned, my other favorite exercise is swimming. Now I know you are going to say, "Well, that's easy for you to say, with your own swimming pool and all." And I cannot deny that Phil and I are very fortunate to be able to afford a private swimming pool at our home. But we earned it—I was a poor kid from the streets of New York, and Phil was a poor kid from the mining country in southern Indiana. Nobody gave us anything, least of all that swimming pool.

Still, it is certainly true that most people do not have a swimming pool in their backyards. So swimming is not as easy for them to do as walking. But it is far from impossible. I know hundreds of people who don't own swimming pools but swim every day. In most communities there is a town pool, or there is a pool at the YMCA, or they open up the high school swimming pool to the townspeople every afternoon. (If they don't, they should; maybe you can start a movement to get the authorities to open up that pool in your hometown.) You may know a neighbor or a friend who has a pool and will let you use it. If you live in an area of lakes, you don't need a pool—the friendly neighborhood lake will do very nicely.

All I'm saying is that you can most likely find someplace where you can swim regularly. And if you do, by all means make a point of doing it. Because next to walking, swimming is the perfect form of exercise. Like walking, it enables you to give every part of your body a good, thorough workout.

If you elect to swim rather than walk—and, of course, you certainly can do both, as I do—you should also keep a chart to record your progress.

I realize some people will say, "Well, I know swimming is a great form of exercise, but there's only one thing wrong with it—I don't know how to swim." All right, for you I'll even change the terminology. I won't call it swimming, I'll call it "water exercise." There are, you see, a lot of exercises that can be done in the water that do not involve actual swimming. The thing is that doing exercises in the water can be more beneficial than doing them on dry land because the water provides some resistance, which means your body has to work that much harder to do the same thing.

For example, you can do the following exercise anywhere, in your den or in a swimming pool: Stand with one hand holding on to a table or the side of the pool and extend your other arm straight out, about shoulder level. Then swing your outside leg out as far as it will go, and bring it back. Then turn around and do the same on the other side.

A good exercise. But it is much better if you do it while standing in the water. As you swing your leg, you have to force it up against the resistance of the water, so that your leg (and you) have to work much harder. As a result, the exercise is considerably more beneficial. That exercise is particularly helpful in firming your legs and thighs. I will ordinarily swim awhile, then go to the side of my pool and do that exercise for perhaps ten minutes.

Next is one that is designed to exercise the arms. Again, you can do it anywhere, but doing it in the water increases its benefits. I stand in the pool, with the water about up to my chest. My feet are apart, my hands at my sides. Then I raise one arm, elbow bent, until it is at chest level, with the palm out. Now I gradually straighten my elbow, pushing the water away until my arm is straight out to the side. It sounds easy, but the resistance of the water is what makes it hard—and valuable. Do that five times with each arm to start with (remember always to stop *before* it begins to hurt), more as your arms grow stronger.

Another great water exercise is simply to hang on to the side of the pool and kick your legs. Ever since we were kids, most of us have gotten a kick out of kicking in water, and making big splashes. I know I have. Well, now you can turn that bit of fun into a beneficial exercise, because if you kick hard enough and long enough you'll get the heart pumping and the blood charging through your veins and arteries and give your legs a workout, too.

While you're at the side of the pool, hanging on, there is another marvelous exercise. Stretch your body out as far as it can go—reach out with your feet as if you were trying to touch something that you could not quite reach. The body benefits from a good stretch like that.

You can add a bit to that by next swinging your legs as wide as they will go, then back to the center. Swing them first to the right, then to the left. Then, for variety's sake, swing one left and one right. It really doesn't matter, because whatever you do in this position is going to be helpful to your body.

In fact, if you are in the water, anything you do is a plus. You can just jump up and down and that's great. Or do a few minutes of dog paddling. Terrific. Or just lie on your back and kick a little. Swell.

That's why I recommend swimming—or rather water exercises—so highly. They don't have to be formal. I have suggested some that you can do, if you want specific exercises. I know some people like to be told exactly what to do. OK, for those people, do the leg exercise for ten minutes, the arm exercise for another ten minutes, and the leg-swinging exercise for the final ten minutes. Then you'll have a half hour of exercising that will benefit every part of your body.

But if you are the kind of person who doesn't want anything that formal, just jump into the pool and horse around for a half hour. If you do it vigorously enough, you will probably get just as much exercise, and derive just as much benefit, as my friend who is doing the exercises by the clock.

And, as you can see, you don't have to know how to swim to do these exercises. If you can hang on to the side of the pool, or to the side of a float if you are in a lake or pond, then you can do my water exercises.

Of course, if you do know how to swim, so much the better. Then you can do these water exercises and/or some regular swimming. The plain old crawl stroke is marvelous. You can vary that with a few laps of breaststroke or, if you really are an expert swimmer, its more modern cousin, the butterfly. The backstroke is also good, and, if all else fails, the good old dog paddle or the sidestroke can't hurt.

So we have you walking and swimming. If you can manage fifteen minutes for walking three times a week, and the same amount of time for swimming, you are doing enough. That hour and a half a week will put you well on the road to good health.

But suppose, for one reason or another, you find it difficult to get out. Perhaps your neighborhood is unsafe, so you are afraid to walk. And maybe you simply cannot find any convenient place to go swimming. Those things happen. I realize not everyone is as fortunate as I am, and not everyone has the opportunity for pleasant walks and pleasant swims. Does that mean you can never exercise, that you are doomed to a sedentary life, with your body growing rotten from not being used properly? Not at all.

If you can breathe, you can do my breathing exercises. If you can stand up, you can do my standing exercises. If you can lie down, you can do my horizontal exercises. There is something for everyone in the Alice Faye system of exercising for Growing Older but Staying Young.

Breathing exercises are important because getting clean air into our lungs is vital to our physical well-being.

I know that the first thing a singing teacher will instruct a new pupil in is the proper way to breathe. Even though I never took a singing lesson in my life, I've talked to enough singers that I know that's the way it goes. Music teachers are convinced, and I am sure they are correct, that most people simply do not know the proper way to breathe. To make sure that your lungs get the best supply of air, and that that supply reaches the deepest crannies of your lungs, you must breathe deeply—from the diaphragm.

So stand on your feet, arms at your sides, and simply take a series of deep breaths. But try to feel your diaphragm pulling the new air in and pushing the old, stale air out. Do this slowly for ten minutes or so.

Another good exercise for your breathing mechanism is to begin again by standing erect with your arms at your sides. Now take a deep breath. Then bend forward at the waist, as if you are taking a bow, and exhale toward the ground, blowing the old, stale air out vigorously. Do that a half dozen times or so.

Standing exercises are essential to keep various parts of your body limber and usable. You know, the body is a marvelous piece of machinery, but, like any piece of machinery, if you don't use it, it will become rusty and cease to function. Keep your car in the garage for six months, and a couple of the parts won't work when you drag it out again. The same holds true for your body. If you don't lift your arm above your head for a protracted period of time—if, say, you break it and it's in a cast—then when you're OK again and want to lift that arm over your head, it will resist. It will take considerable effort to get that arm up where you want it. And some poor souls, through such inactivity, permanently lose the ability to move one of their joints through its intended range of motion.

It happens all the time. You see some older people who simply can no longer move their arms above their heads, or bend their elbows completely, or bend at the waist. Through inactivity they have lost the use of a joint, partially or sometimes totally. And that loss was unnecessary. I know an expert in this field who says the motto of everyone over fifty should be Use It or Lose It.

The thing you have to try to do is put your joints through that entire range of movement at least once a day. That isn't a difficult thing to do, and it doesn't take long. Here's how to do it, in a form I call my standing exercises.

First, for your neck—don't forget, your neck is a kind of joint, and you need to keep it exercised and limber. Stand straight and simply turn your head to the right, then to the left, as far as it will go. See if you can look behind you—if you can, your neck is good and limber. If you can't, try to do a little more each day until you can.

Next, your shoulders. Again, start from a standing position. Now make believe you are swimming. The crawl, of course. Take your right arm; swing it back and down and then up and around and forward. Just as if you were in the water. Then do the same with your left arm. Continue, alternating arms, while you swim several laps across the living room, or wherever it is you are doing the exercise. Your shoulders are going through their normal, full range of motion that way.

One of the best exercises I know of for helping the shoulders is this: Stand with your feet apart. Now bend your body to the left and lift your right arm as high and as far over your head to the left as it will go. Then do this in the other direction, bending to the right and lifting your arm up and across, over your head.

Your hips need some exercising, too. Anybody who has ever had problems with his or her hips knows how painful it can be if that important joint acts up. So be sure to include some exercises that give the hips a workout.

Here's one: Stand with your feet apart, on your toes. Pivot on your right foot, twisting right, until you are looking directly down at your right heel. Then twist a little more! Do the same thing in the other direction. This exercise not only puts your hips to the test but is a good stretch for your back muscles, too.

The knees are one of our most vulnerable joints, as any athlete or dancer will attest. So in any exercise regimen, you should pay particular attention to the knees. This is my favorite exercise to give the knees a workout: Stand straight, with your hands on your hips. Now step and lunge forward, bending your right knee. Then do the same with your left knee. Continue, alternating knees, several times.

Of course, the good old deep knee bend is the classic

exercise for the knees. In case you have forgotten that standby of the high school gym teacher, you stand with your hands on your hips, then simply bend your knees and let your body go down, slowly, trying to keep your back straight as you go. Very good for the knees, the back, and the muscles in your legs.

Another of my favorite standing exercises is one that involves pretty much the entire body. Start out, once more, standing erect, with your feet slightly apart. Now try to touch your right foot with your left hand, beginning by swinging your arm up and back and then down and toward the ground. Then do the reverse—try to touch your left foot with your right hand. Keep alternating, right hand, left hand, for several minutes.

In this exercise, and in any exercise that asks you to bend over, don't try to be a hero and keep your legs straight. If you force your legs to remain stiff and straight, you are putting a lot of undue strain on your back, and it could go out on you, like that. Bend your knees a little; nobody is watching, and even if someone is, so what? It's your back, not theirs.

Another standing exercise, out of the old high school gym class repertoire, is the jumping jack. Surely you remember that one? It used to be the bane of my life. You start out with your arms at your sides, then you jump up and push your legs out and, simultaneously, swing your arms up and clap hands over your head. Then jump up, put your feet back in place, and do it again. I remember we had to do that one over and over, until I just about dropped. But it is still a good exercise, for the legs and the arms and the shoulders and, of course, the heart and the circulatory system. I usually wind up my session of standing exercises with ten or twelve jumping jacks.

You can also get a good workout simply by running in place. Or, if you want to really go back to your childhood, a little skipping rope. (We didn't know it when we were kids on the sidewalks of New York, but those rope-skipping games we played were terrific exercises.)

The last group of exercises are the horizontal exercises. All you need for these is a convenient floor. And your body. You can even do them on the bed, if it is impossible for you to get up and about, but, of course, the floor is preferable.

The best is that old-fashioned torture mechanism the sit-up. Simply begin in a lying-down position and then sit up. Sounds easy, but it makes strong men weep. The object, of course, is to sit up without lifting your legs. Obviously, we young elders are allowed to cheat a little. Even with the cheating, though, this is a difficult exercise and one that is good for the entire body. You have to bend your knees a bit, of course. Otherwise, you could hurt your back.

Another horizontal exercise requires you to get on your hands and knees. Begin with your head down. Then stretch your right leg as far back as it will go, while you lift your head up as high as it will go. Then the left leg. This one is great for your back, neck, and leg muscles.

One more horizontal exercise. Lie on your back for this one and bring both legs up as high as possible, maybe until your feet are directly above your head.

A variation on this is the horizontal bicycle. Again lying on your back, bring both legs up and pretend you are pedaling an imaginary bicycle. Keep pedaling until you reach Albuquerque or you get tired, whichever comes first.

There is another horizontal exercise that I call the "leg touch." Start lying flat on your back. Now bring your left arm back, over your head. Try to keep your back flat on the ground (or floor, or bed, or mat, or Oriental rug, or whatever it is you're lying on). Now simultaneously lift both your left leg and your left arm and try to touch them. Don't force it, of course—in exercising, never force yourself to go further than is comfortable—but do the best you can. Then try the same thing with your right leg and right arm. This works wonders for your back and tummy.

I do one exercise from the horizontal position that I call "superstretch." Starting from a prone position, bring both knees up until they are as close to your chest as you can manage. Clasp your hands around your legs, about at your shins. Now let go with the right hand and extend your right leg forward until it is straight and almost touching the floor (or grass or braided rug or whatever). At the same time, bring your right arm back over your head until it is practically touching the floor (or parquet or weeds or whatever). You are stretching one way with your leg and the other way with your arm. Now bring both arm and leg back to the original position and hug them tight to your chest.

Now do the same thing, this time using your left leg and left arm. Remember to stretch as far as you can without dislocating something or other. This is a marvelous way to exercise those tired stomach muscles—and, who knows, you might grow an inch or two.

I also like an exercise I call the "rollover." Flat on your back again, gang. Now keep your left leg straight out, but bring your right leg up, until your right foot is resting lightly on your left thigh, with the knee bent and pointing skyward. Throw your arms out wide, until they are touching the ground with the palms down. Here comes the hard part—roll that right leg as far to the left as you can, while trying to keep those arms flat on the ground. While the leg is over as far as it will go, bounce it up and down—gently—a few times. Now roll back to the original position and do the exercise again, only this time going the other way.

The last of my horizontal exercises is the "knee roll." Lie on your back and bring your knees up, as close to your chest as you can without breaking anything. Put your hands on your waist, with your elbows touching the floor. Now roll both of your knees to the left, then push your feet straight out, diagonally, to the left. Now, with the legs still pointing in that direction, bend your knees again and roll back to the starting position. Do the same exercise going in the other direction. If you can do that six times each way you will soon be very healthy—and very tired. But you will feel great!

There are, of course, hundreds of other exercises you can do. I only mean to suggest a few here. The important thing is to do something, even if it is only—as Phil often says, but I think he is only joking—a little card shuffling and dealing.

Some people say they don't have time for exercise, they are just too busy and can't be bothered. To them, I would like to relay this suggestion from an old wardrobe lady at Fox. I had to dash into the ladies' room at the commissary one day, and there was this dear old lady, hanging on to the sink and doing some deep knee bends.

"What on earth are you doing, Laura?" I asked her.

"Oh, Miss Faye," she said, "I'm doing my exercises. I like to keep myself in shape, but I haven't got time for any real exercises, so whenever I go to the bathroom, I do this for about five minutes or so."

Thinking back on Laura and her five minutes whenever she went to the bathroom, I realize it's not such a bad idea. How many times do you go to the bathroom each day? Probably five or six. Doing a five-minute session of exercises every time—and holding on to the sink is a good way of doing them—gives you a half hour or so of workout. Yet you don't feel as though you've actually spent a half hour exercising. You have just stolen a few minutes here and there.

Another way of outnegotiating yourself is to do some exercising in bed. Make it ten minutes before you get up and another ten just when you climb in at night. A few exercises for you in bed—stretching up and back, then down to try to touch your toes; crossing over, bringing your right arm down to your left foot and vice versa; sitting up from a prone position. Incidentally, if you are confined to bed for any reason, these are good exercises to do so you don't get too far behind in your exercise program.

I know people who believe that the best form of exercise is bicycling. No question about it, it is terrific. I just feel that for me, and for most young elders, it is a little too strenuous. Too much of a good thing. The same with aerobics. Without a doubt, it does wonders for a body. Look at Jane Fonda. But you have to be young and in pretty good shape to start with, or aerobics can be very harmful. Going to a gym for a heavy workout can also make one slim and trim—but if you don't know what you're doing, it can make you a very banged-up, unhealthy individual. That stuff is mostly for kids or professional athletes.

Moreover, all of the above—bicycling, aerobics, workouts at a gym—cost money, one way or another. Walking is free, and so are the exercises I've just suggested (you might want to invest in a mat for your bedroom—a bit softer than the floor—perhaps an exercise outfit, but neither of those are musts). You may have to pay for the use of a swimming pool, but maybe not. Even if you do, the cost is probably nominal.

All it costs to walk, to exercise, is a little effort, and a bit of willpower. And it is worth every bit of that effort, that willpower. It is entirely up to you. If you don't want to do it, nobody is going to put a gun to your head and make you. You alone have to reach the decision that you should do it.

If you have easy access to a swimming pool, as I do with my own pool just outside my back door, I suggest you jump in a few times a day. That's what I do. I actually go into my pool four or five times every single day when I'm home. In the Palm Springs area, where I live, the weather is seldom too cold for a dip. I find if I don't swim for several minutes, several times a day, I miss it very badly. My body seems to feel the lack of that particular form of exercise. On chilly days I do other things—the exercises I outlined earlier—but I really believe that water exercises are, for me at least, the ultimate form of exercise next to walking.

I want to stress here that it doesn't matter how old you are—or how young you are. You are never either too young or too old to begin exercising on a regular basis. I know from my children and grandchildren—and from my own experience, too—that young people often think exercising is a silly thing to do. And for many young people who lead active lives, it is superfluous. Still, it is a great habit to get into. I realize it is hard for young people to think they will ever get old, but it happens to a lot of us. And if you get into the exercising habit when you are young, you can segue into the older years, when you desperately need exercise, without so much as losing a beat. Even if you find yourself in your sixties or seventies, and you have never so much as bent a knee in pursuit of exercise, it is not too late to start. It will be harder, of course, but far from impossible.

Exercise will, no matter what your age or previous condition of physique, improve the flexibility in your joints and muscles, and that will, of course, make it easier to do the little things around the house that can sometimes be painful and difficult. And walking and swimming will better your muscle tone.

I am told by my doctor friends that recent research seems to indicate that exercise may also result in an increase in bone mass. That, they tell me, can be very important to people who suffer from osteoporosis.

Brisk walking and brisk swimming, since they get the heart pumping and the blood circulating, can be very beneficial to your overall state of cardiovascular fitness as well. This means a reduced risk of stroke, heart disease, and such. (It can also help you lose weight, if this is something you desire.)

There seems to be no question in the scientific community that a definite correlation exists between exercising and longevity. I remember reading about one study that compared the life span of two groups of men. One group regularly had to walk up a long flight of stairs to get to work. The other didn't. And the stair-climbing men lived considerably longer.

I want to reiterate here what I said earlier about checking with your doctor before beginning any regular exercise program. I can't stress that too often. No matter what you read in some magazine, or hear on television or the radio, advocating that you do this series of exercises or that, please ask your personal physician about it before you begin. Your own medical history may be such that those exercises would actually do you more harm than good.

One other word of caution, which may be unnecessary, but I feel I must say it. I have urged walking. But I want to suggest that women should be very careful before they go walking about at night. There are a lot of weird people abroad in this world, and women have to be extremely cautious. But you can always find a safe place and a safe time for a walk.

Or a swim.

Or my exercises.

The key is to do something. And to do it on a regular basis. And, further, to increase the amount of time you do the walking, swimming, and/or exercising. (Increase it only up to a certain amount of time, however; after a while a point of diminishing returns sets in, and the additional time you work out does not give additional benefit.)

One last point about exercising. If at all possible, do it outdoors. Walking, I find, is much more pleasurable in an outdoor setting, although I know a lot of people who walk around shopping malls. The problem there is the temptation to window-shop, which limits the value of exercise. Still, I don't knock it—but try to keep your eyes straight ahead. And even my other exercises can be done outside, weather permitting. And they should be done outside, if you can, because you get an extra added benefit from being out-of-doors.

I think most of us have always been told, since we were children, that being outside is good for you. But we probably never were told why—maybe because our parents had never been told themselves, and therefore had no idea why.

Lately, scientific studies have pinpointed the value of the out-of-doors. There may be more than one value, but the one that made the biggest impression on me came in a recent report by the former surgeon general of the United States, Dr. C. Everett Koop. This report says that exposure to the sun aids the body in its efforts to absorb calcium. A person who drinks a glass of milk but stays indoors will, the report indicates, get less benefit from that milk than a person who drinks the same quantity but then goes out and basks in the sunshine.

The report suggests that exposure to the sun for ten to fifteen minutes, two or three times a week, is adequate. Of course, you have to balance that suggestion against other advice about too much sun causing a danger of skin cancer. I personally think that you can get enough sun outside, indirectly, without feeling you have to lie in the sun's direct rays. I am outside a lot—walking, swimming—and I believe I get my quota of sunshine that way. It's pleasanter, too, to exercise outside when the weather is nice.

Exercise, then, is the first step in Growing Older but Staying Young.

The next step is your diet.

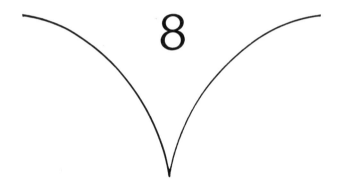

8

Nutrition is an inexact science, if it can be dignified by being called a science in the first place. Some sciences—such as chemistry or mathematics—are exact and precise; A is always A and B is always B. But not nutrition.

You can talk to Nutritionist Smith, and he will tell you that eggs are terrible, being so full of that nasty old cholesterol. Then you pick up a book by Nutritionist Jones and read that eggs are the perfect food, and a little cholesterol is good for you. One will say take loads of vitamins, another will say too many vitamins can hurt you. And the same for other foods and other diets. The nutritionists seem to be in the business of contradicting each other. So what is a body to do?

My solution, and, as I said earlier, I am reasonably healthy and my weight hasn't varied much in nearly sixty years, is to do what I was taught as a kid: Eat a balanced diet. But don't eat too much of it.

It seems to me that this is extremely sensible advice. The main thing to remember, when you think about what to put in your stomach, is what we human beings are. We are animals, mammals, carnivores, and our bodies are built so that we need the same kind of foods that other animals, mammals, carnivores need. So fad diets—such as vegetarianism, or the grapefruit diet, or any of those kooky diets in those kooky diet books from those kooky diet experts—are bad for our systems if we stick to them for too long. Our bodies need a variety of things, and it's up to us to feed ourselves intelligently.

Many people are chiefly concerned with losing weight. There is no question that excess poundage is a serious problem in the world today. Just look around you, and you'll see so many people who are terribly overweight, to the point of obesity.

Not only is that unattractive, it is very unhealthy.

Science has proved that a link exists between being overweight and several serious health conditions:

Obesity can be a contributory cause of heart disease.
Obesity can be a contributory cause of strokes.
Obesity can be a contributory cause of high blood pressure.
Obesity can be a contributory cause of diabetes.

And recent research indicates clearly that what we eat can also help cause certain types of cancer. In fact, roughly one-third of all cancers are traceable to dietary problems, mostly diets consisting of too much fat and not enough fiber.

So we would all be smart to keep our weight down. I know people will say, "That's easy for her to say—she's always been thin." True, but I believe that if I didn't watch what I eat, I could very easily turn into a baby balloon. When I was a young girl, back before I became a professional dancer, I had what we used to call "kid fat." (That's the same thing as "baby fat," only a few years older.) If I hadn't started dancing just then, and thus embarked on a forced regimen of exercise that kept my weight down, I think I might have become a genuinely fat person.

There are very few people who never have to worry about their weight. And they are primarily anorexics and others who have weight problems in reverse—they want to put some weight on their skinny frames. But the majority of people, at some point in their lives, have to watch it, or they will blimp up.

There are all kinds of diets, all sorts of food plans. You can waste your money on high-cost, low-calorie foods at the supermarket. You can take pills to control your appetite. You can endanger your health (and your pocketbook) with dangerous and expensive products such as liquid protein. You can buy diet books until your bookshelves are bulging. And chances are your stomach will still be bulging, too.

Actually, the answer is very simple: Eat whatever you want, just eat less of it.

There is an old bit of doggerel that I've always felt is so appropriate to this issue:

If you want to lose some weight
Simply push away the plate.

My theory is that, as a general rule, people eat too much. We don't need all the food we cram into our stomachs. We eat enough to keep our bodies going and satisfy our hunger—and then we eat more. Most people seem to be always stuffing something into their mouths.

They eat breakfast. Then, midmorning, they stop for a little bite of something or other. Then it's lunchtime. And often they punctuate their afternoons with a candy bar around two-thirty and an ice cream cone around four. Then, before dinner, they have some cheese and crackers with their cocktails. Next comes dinner, and later, while watching TV, they nibble on bowls of potato chips or candy. Then, just before bedtime, they fix themselves a nice fat sandwich and drink a bottle of beer.

They have eaten something nine times during the day. That's six more times than is necessary. They haven't eaten to satisfy their hunger. They have eaten just for the sake of eating.

Some people eat and grow fat, then diet themselves back to normal, then go on an eating binge and it's back up twenty-five pounds or so. And they repeat the cycle, over and over again. They laugh about it, about how they have a fat wardrobe and a skinny wardrobe and go from one to the other four or five times a year. It's become a way of life. It is also a very unhealthy way of life, because such fluctuations actually put an undue strain on the body. Just when your body adjusts to carrying around one weight, and supplying that weight with blood and oxygen and such, you go on a diet and the body has to make major adjustments in its supply system.

If you can take weight off, you should keep it off. I realize that is easier said than done, but it can be done—if you simply push the plate away. If you do that, you can eat your favorite foods. The sacrifice you are making is merely one of quantity, not quality. Eat the whole range of rich, gloppy foods you want—but less of them.

I will always remember reading about Judy Garland who, when she was a teenager, had Louis B. Mayer on her case about her weight. The poor thing, at that time in her life, was a very healthy girl, but she was one of those kids who looked at a piece of cake and gained six pounds. The movie camera, of course, makes anybody look heavier, so Mayer hounded her and hounded her to lose weight and she tried. But she lost so much energy that the studio gave her pep-up pills that were, I believe, the beginning of her problems. All through her life she went from being too fat to being much too thin, and she would take pills for each condition. Finally she became so totally addicted to pills that they did her in. That's the danger in what I call the artificial road to weight control. I strongly advocate the opposite—the natural way.

I believe one major problem with most diets is that they fail to take into consideration one very important element— the factor of individual taste. We are all different in so many ways, and one of those ways is that we all like some foods and dislike others. I happen to be crazy about pasta. Phil says he thinks I must have some Italian blood, to go with my Irish and German heritage, because of the way I can gobble up pasta. So any diet that allows me pasta would, in my book, be a good diet. Similarly, I would be unhappy with a diet that was totally pasta free.

That's why my system works for everybody. I eat pasta whenever I want—I just limit how much I eat. I still love pasta, despite what happened one day when I was making a movie called *You Can't Have Everything*. According to the script, I was supposed to eat a big bowl of spaghetti. Take after take I ate spaghetti, and finally, as a gag, Don Ameche, my costar, had the director, Norman Taurog, make believe the take was bad. I kept shoveling spaghetti down while the cast and crew tried not to laugh. I must have eaten fifteen bowls of spaghetti that day.

If you like meat and potatoes, eat meat and potatoes— but keep the portions small. Have cake or pie or ice cream for dessert, just keep the slices tiny, or at least less big than you have been used to giving yourself.

Think about it logically. If you have always dished yourself out portions that were, say, x big, and now, using my plan, you cut those portions by a quarter, naturally you will be eating a quarter fewer calories. You don't have to count calories, just cut your serving down by a certain percentage to cut your calories by that same percentage. I don't expect you to take a ruler or a scale and measure things on your plate. Just estimate roughly how big your portions have traditionally been and cut them by enough to make a difference.

As I said, I had kid fat before I started dancing. Then, when I began my movie career, there were still some vestiges of that condition, particularly around my face. The studio brass, beginning with Darryl Zanuck, passed the word down to me that I was a bit too "chubby." That was a nice way of saying that I was on the verge of being fat. And, they added, I had better do something about it. And fast, if I wanted to stay under contract. So I did something about it. And fast. I began eating less.

In one way I was very lucky. My extra weight was in a place—my face—where it came off easily and quickly. I'd always had thin legs, and that's where extra weight is very hard to shed. But I cut down on my food intake, and within a few weeks my face was thinner and I never again heard any complaints from the studio hierarchy about my weight.

I was lucky in another way, too. That system of studio supervision stood me in good stead then. They supervised my diet until I had slimmed down to the point where their supervision was no longer necessary. So for those few weeks I ate an awful lot of cottage cheese and grilled lamb chops. Today I don't care if I never see another dollop of cottage cheese or another lamb chop, with or without its paper panties.

From then on, I began habitually to quit eating while I could still eat some more. It isn't that I am exactly hungry, just that I am not overfull. There is a big difference. And I have trained my stomach, and my mind, to be entirely satisfied with what I give myself. I could probably eat more, but I have gotten into the habit of quitting while I'm still just the slightest bit hungry. I think you will find that after a month or so you will get used to that condition.

So it doesn't matter so much what you eat; what matters is how much of it you eat. Look at Audrey Hepburn. She's a pasta girl, like myself. She once said that pasta is basically all she ever eats. Nobody could ever accuse Audrey of being fat, yet pasta is considered a fattening food. I assume that, like me, she'll eat pasta but do two things to militate against its caloric content:

1. Eat small portions.

2. Watch what she puts on top of the pasta, and what she eats with it.

I know a lot of people who wouldn't think of eating spaghetti without some garlic bread on the side. And, of course, a great ocean of rich, fattening sauce on top. This way disaster lies. You really don't need bread with your pasta; the pasta alone is sufficient. And there are many ways I serve pasta without that heavy layer of calories that calls itself spaghetti sauce.

In fact, my very favorite pasta dish is this: Cook a pot of pasta—spaghetti or fettuccine or whatever happens to be your pet—as you would ordinarily cook your pasta. Then drain it, empty a can of chicken broth over it, and add a whole mess of chopped green onions. I use the low-fat chicken broth, too. (Thank Heaven that we live in this enlightened era of low-fat foods!)

This is absolutely delicious. I am also very partial to old-fashioned macaroni and cheese. That is a bit more fattening, so I eat a little less of it. But I could literally eat pasta at every meal and be a happy person. I don't, of course, because as I said earlier I am a firm believer in a balanced diet.

I believe one advantage I possess is that I have a strong stomach. I can put just about anything in it without suffering any digestive problems. My poor husband, however, has a stomach of a different color. He gets indigestion at the drop of a pizza. He chews antacid pills like some people chew gum.

One reason, I believe, that my stomach is so well behaved is the training I gave it when I was a young woman. Back in those days, when I was on the road with Rudy Vallee's band

and doing all sorts of one-nighters, I was forced to eat horribly. I would eat at all hours of the day or night, whenever I had the chance, and I would eat wherever I happened to be. Mostly, that was in some greasy spoon diner around the corner from the ballroom where I was singing, and I would generally order a fried egg sandwich. At least when you have an egg you can be pretty sure it comes out of a shell; with anything else in those places it is a gastronomical gamble.

I survived a few thousand late night and early morning fried egg sandwiches. Somehow. And my stomach learned to take what I was forced to give it and digest it and never grumble about it. It's amazing what your stomach can take when you are young. I think those years of wild and woolly eating made my stomach impervious to harm.

However, I realize there are millions of people who do have problems with their digestive systems. Obviously, these people should eat bland, easily digestible foods. But these foods can be fattening, too, so even people eating them should follow my lead of getting up from the table *before* they eat too much.

Even though I can eat anything, I think I eat sensibly. My theory is that the body needs a little bit of a lot of things. A balanced diet, as I have said, is very important.

I have talked to many nutritionists, doctors, dieticians, and others who are knowledgeable about what we should and should not eat. I have also read dozens of books on the subject. While there are often areas of disagreement about some things, there are broad areas where all the experts agree. And I have synthesized the information I have gotten from these discussions and my reading and have come up with what I believe every human body needs in the way of food.

A balanced diet should consist of food from five groups: grain products, vegetables, fruit, dairy products, and protein-rich foods such as meat, fish, and certain other foods. Those are the standard food groups, but I add a sixth, not so much for its nutritional value as for its psychological value.

That sixth group is one I call "treats." My point here is that if you eat well and follow my advice about not overeating, then once in a while you can give yourself a treat—a slice of lemon meringue pie or a piece of chocolate.

There is no way a treat once a week is going to harm you, but it could do you a world of mental good. If you are one of those people who crave something sweet, and you believe your diet is condemning you to a life without such a treat forevermore, then you will have great difficulty sticking with it. But if you know you are permitted to indulge yourself once in a while, then it will be considerably easier on you to stay with the other parts of your diet.

Let us look at these six basic food groups more closely.

GRAIN PRODUCTS: This group includes my favorite, pasta, plus breads, cereals, rice, and even grain-based products such as pancakes, waffles, scones, and muffins.

I have no intention of telling you how much of what you should or can eat. I only want to say that, to be balanced, your diet should include something from this group every day. Not necessarily at every meal, but every day.

VEGETABLES: I have heard experts say that you should eat three (or two or four or how ever many) different vegetables a day. I don't think we have to be slaves to counting the number of different vegetables we eat, any more than we have to be slaves to counting calories. But it stands to reason that we should eat different vegetables because each one has its own assortment of vitamins and other stuff that is good for you.

Certainly we all know, and we always have known since Mommy told us to eat up all our peas, that vegetables are good for us. So the balanced diet should include vegetables every day, and, if you can vary them, that's beneficial.

I have heard that the darker the color of the vegetable,

the more nutrition it contains. Thus, among yellow vegetables the dark yellow winter squash is more nutritious than pale yellow wax beans. And broccoli is more nutritious than those light green baby peas. This principle seems to make sense to me, so I try to have some dark-hued vegetables every day.

FRUIT: An apple a day, et cetera. This may be just an old wives' saying, but if that wife is old enough, maybe she still makes some sense. Certainly there is no doubt in anybody's mind that a piece of fruit is a healthy thing to eat, and a good, sensible alternative to that candy bar so many people crave.

Fruit should be in your balanced diet, and again a variety of fruits is better than just one, because each sort contains different good things. As with vegetables, you should bear in mind that the darker the color, the more healthful—so, for example, a piece of deep yellow melon is supposedly more full of nutrition than a slice of pale yellow pineapple.

Most of us have long believed that we should start the day with a glass of orange juice. So full of vitamin C, we have always been told. And that is true—but orange juice is not the only good source of vitamin C. There are alternatives, if you get a little bored with the same old orange juice every morning. Strawberries are supposed to be just as vitamin C–full as orange juice, and cantaloupe is another fruit that has more than its share of that helpful vitamin. So you can vary your balanced diet by having strawberries or cantaloupe occasionally.

DAIRY PRODUCTS: The well-balanced diet should include one or two items from the dairy group every day. Milk, of course, heads the list, but I realize a lot of people don't like milk. I prefer to get my dairy product in the form of yogurt, which is just as healthful and, to me, a lot better tasting. You can also supply your body with the dairy product it needs in the form of some kind of cheese—from cottage through cream to the more substantial ones, such as cheddar, Swiss, or Muenster. Any old cheese will do. But you have to have some form of dairy product in your daily diet.

I don't much like whole milk. Never have. Not since I was a child have I willingly had a glass of milk. Yet I know the stuff is good for me. Actually, as we grow older, we need more calcium. Youngsters need calcium—a prime ingredient in bone structure—when their bones are being built. And in our later years we need it again, to keep those bones from becoming brittle and breakable.

I have seen tables of RDAs—recommended daily allowances—for many items, and the RDA for milk for people in my age bracket is 800 milligrams. A glass of skim milk (we won't even talk regular milk) has 300 milligrams. So you can see that three glasses of milk a day and you're over the requirement. But suppose you are like me, and a glass of milk never touches your lips. How, then, do you get your calcium? Cheese is a good source; so is yogurt. So are calcium pills, but many doctors believe it is better to get your calcium naturally. I feel that I get enough here and there, with a cup of yogurt from time to time, some Parmesan cheese strewn cheerfully over my pasta, and the occasional grilled cheese sandwich.

PROTEIN-RICH FOOD: Heading the list of protein-rich foods is, of course, meat. I realize that red meat has acquired a bad reputation these days, and most experts seem to agree that the average American has long been eating too much beef, too many steaks and chops. Incidentally, as proof of how health-conscious America has become, there is this telling statistic from the U.S. Department of Agriculture: In 1970 the annual per capita consumption of red meat in America was 131.9 pounds; that declined, in the ensuing fifteen years, by more than 10.0 pounds, and at the same time the consumption of fish and poultry products went up by a similar amount.

So we are eating less red meat, and that is probably a good thing—but I don't think it is right to eliminate red meat from our diets entirely. Every once in a while I will crave a steak or a nice juicy slice of roast beef. I think that craving is my body telling me it needs some red meat.

So the balanced diet should include some red meat, I think. Perhaps once a week. And plenty of poultry and fish. You can substitute other foods for meat, poultry, or fish at some meals. Some beans—such as black beans or kidney beans, lentils or lima beans—are excellent sources of protein, too. They also give you the fiber your diet should have.

But I believe it is wrong to attempt to get all of our protein from these other sources. There are some things in the meat, poultry, and fish that a bean cannot supply—maybe it is the fact that we humans are meat-eating mammals, and so, perhaps in our subconscious, there is the need to eat flesh. At any rate, I believe that some meat is essential for the well-balanced diet. Not a lot, but some.

Finally, that sixth category I have added—the treat. Now there is nothing scientific about this, merely my hunch that a treat now and then is good for the soul, and you have to keep your soul as well nourished as your body. So, maybe once a week, reward yourself for being a good girl (or boy) with a nice dessert or some candy.

I am fortunate in that I don't have a particularly sweet tooth. But once in a while I like a piece of chocolate. (And I do have one quirk—when I fly, I always nibble on M & M's. These days, the food on most planes is bad, so I carry my M & M's to give me strength, sustenance, and maybe even courage.)

But I very seldom indulge in dessert of any kind. It simply is something I got out of the habit of doing long ago, and these days I truly don't miss it. Habits, you know, can be good or bad, and there is a habit of eating a particular kind of food—such as dessert—and there is also a habit of not eating it.

I know dessert eaters will scoff and say they could never stop eating desserts. But if you just don't have them around the house for a few weeks, so you couldn't eat dessert even if you wanted to, before you know it the good habit—of not eating dessert—will have superseded the bad habit—of eating dessert. That's what happened to me, and, as I say, nowadays I get up from the table, dessertless, and don't even think about it. It's habitual to have no dessert.

Another bad habit many of us have gotten into is the snack. At any hour of day or night, people nibble. A few potato chips here, a candy bar there, ice cream, cookies, whatever. It all adds up, in calories and fat and other bad things, and pretty soon the weight begins to climb. Snacking is a caloric calamity.

Don't eat between meals.

But if you simply must nibble on something, choose popcorn. It is the least harmful of all the recognized snacking foods—provided, of course, that you don't drench it in butter or shower it with salt—and, although it contains little of nutritional value, it also contains little that is harmful.

Some people stop in their day's activities from time to time to eat a carton of yogurt. Or they use yogurt as their entire luncheon menu. Yogurt is a very fine food. As we get older its value increases, because, as I said earlier, one of its components is a high percentage of calcium. So there are those who say that an occasional yogurt snack shouldn't be considered bad. I still feel that it is an indulgence to eat between meals, and that yogurt, despite its beneficial side, does contain some calories, which you don't need. Use yogurt as a breakfast or lunch food, or, as some people do—particularly with the delicious fruit-flavored yogurts that are now available—as a dessert at dinnertime.

I stick to three meals a day. Period.

To those who simply must have something in between—have a drink of water. It is surprising how water can take the edge off the appetite. Moreover, we really should drink a lot of water every day. We need the lubrication that water gives to our skin, and we need the value water gives to our internal system. My doctor, and most doctors, suggests we drink six glasses a day.

You might be interested in the daily schedule in the Harris household:

I'm usually up and about every morning around seven. As I have said, Phil likes to sleep in longer than I do, but he usually manages to push himself out of bed about a half hour later. So I wait until he is up before I eat breakfast. In the meantime, I'll take the two poodles out for a walk if the weather permits, and it usually does in the Coachella Valley, where we live.

I come back and fix our breakfast. We are big on oatmeal. If it is too hot for hot cereal, we go for a boxed cereal, something like corn flakes or Total. Phil will usually have orange juice, but I prefer other fruits—a piece of melon or an orange or a grapefruit from one of our own trees. (It's very nice to be able to go outside, pick an orange or a grapefruit, and come in and eat it right away.) In the summer I dearly love a piece of watermelon to start the day off right.

I also have a cup of tea. I very seldom will drink coffee, not for any reason except that I don't particularly like it. I do believe, however, that many people drink much too much coffee. It is addictive—caffeine is a drug, after all—and it stands to reason that anything done to excess cannot fail but be hurtful. I add some honey and low-fat milk to my tea, and we use low-fat milk on our cereal, too. No sugar, however, on anything.

So that's my usual breakfast—fruit, cereal, tea.

I am a great lunch person. I love lunch. It is, perhaps, my favorite meal of the entire day.

Generally, I eat lunch early—about 11:30 or so—because I have usually done a lot of physical things in the morning. I have gone for a long walk and jumped into the pool a time or two. So I am hungry by 11:30. My lunch menu varies considerably. I will often have pasta in one form or another. If I do have pasta, I don't eat any bread with it. I don't happen to be a particularly avid salad eater, although once in a while I will make myself a salad. I guess my aversion to salad goes back to those days at the studio, when Darryl Zanuck's edict came down that I had to be careful about my weight, so I almost always had cottage cheese and sliced tomatoes for lunch. So my lunch may be pasta, occasionally a salad or some kind of sandwich. And, usually, a glass of iced tea.

We eat our main meal in the evening. We usually have dinner around seven, or even a bit before. I think it is hard on people to eat a late dinner and then toddle off to bed with all that food in their stomachs. It makes it tough on the digestive tract, and I think that very well may be one reason so many people have problems sleeping. I don't like to go to bed with a full stomach, so we eat early and go to bed empty and sleep like babies.

Our dinners are relatively light, too. A main course of chicken or fish or, perhaps once a week, red meat. A vegetable. Potatoes of some kind, or perhaps pasta or rice. A small green salad to go with it. And that's about it. No appetizer. No dessert. And, the most important thing, the portions are small. I get up from the table feeling satisfied but not over-stuffed.

And certainly nothing more after dinner. We watch television in the evening, but there is no candy box open by my chair and we don't rush to the refrigerator during the commercial breaks to dish ourselves bowls of ice cream.

That's it for the day—breakfast, lunch, dinner.

I have talked to enough doctors, whose opinions I respect, to have learned a few things about what to eat and what not to eat. As I said earlier, you can always find a nutritionist to contradict what another nutritionist has said, but there does seem to be a unanimity of opinion about certain things.

Everybody agrees, apparently, that whole grain breads are more nutritious than white bread, even if it is enriched. So we eat the dark breads—whole wheat, cracked wheat, rye, pumpernickel. And, again, once you get used to that—once you get into a good habit—you find that you don't miss white bread at all.

I try to eat foods that contain fiber. Doctors today are agreed that a high fiber diet does reduce the risk of getting certain types of cancer—particularly cancer of the colon or of the rectum. Foods that are high in fiber include fruits, vegetables, potatoes, breads (whole grain ones again), and dried peas and beans.

At the same time you add fiber to your diet, you should try to eliminate, as much as possible, things like sugar, salt, and fats. Sugar, in excess, is bad for the teeth; it's also high in calories and low in minerals and vitamins. If you can't eat without a sweetener, there are today several artificial sweeteners that add sweetness without adding peril to the diet.

Salt—sodium—is believed to be a major cause of high blood pressure. There are salt substitutes today, too, but try eating your food without extra seasoning—pepper is OK—and soon you will find that you don't miss salt at all.

Fats are another suspected culprit in causing cancers, particularly cancer of the breast in women and cancer of the prostate in men, as well as colon or rectal cancer in everybody. So avoid deep-fried foods and oil-rich salad dressings. Trim your meat of all excess fat before you eat it. You know which foods are fatty, so steer clear of them.

Cholesterol is one of today's scare topics, but, from what

I have heard from my doctor friends, the jury is still out as far as what actual harm that substance does. Many people who eat diets chock-full of cholesterol never have any problems because of it. Others, who consume only small amounts, do have problems. There are drugs that minimize the effect of cholesterol, but it is, of course, better to eliminate the substance from your diet as much as possible if your doctor tells you you should.

Some research lately, I am told, shows that material made from the husks of psyllium seeds can cut down cholesterol in your body by as much as 15 percent. Now most of us don't have a ready supply of psyllium seeds, and even if we did we wouldn't be about to husk the little rascals. But a commercial product called Metamucil contains this material and—if your doctor agrees—can be used as a way of cutting down your cholesterol. Another food that is useful in controlling cholesterol is oat bran; this finding is making America's cereal manufacturers ecstatic. Still, the surest way of reducing the cholesterol in your body is to cut out foods—such as egg yolks, milk, cheese, red meat—that are high in cholesterol. But, as always, check with your doctor first.

Drinking too much alcohol is another risky thing. We have all heard—and it appears to be true—that too much alcohol can cause cirrhosis of the liver, a fatal disease. But research in recent years has indicated that alcohol can also be a cause of cancer—cancer of the mouth, the throat, or the liver. And apparently the risk of this goes up if the drinker is also a heavy smoker. Furthermore, alcoholic drinks are high in calories and correspondingly low in anything of nutritional value.

No matter how healthfully you eat, you won't cure any diseases you may already have. Even the most ardent nutritionist doesn't claim that good nutrition heals or cures. What it can do, however, is ease certain symptoms of certain diseases. It can also give your body strength, so you don't have to take so much medication. And there are increasing indications that good eating habits can prevent the onset of certain diseases.

For many people, the word "diet" implies losing weight, or trying to. Obviously, shedding a few pounds is a major concern of thousands of people. And there are thousands of others who kid themselves along and say that they really don't have a weight problem at all. They are the ones who, when they can't squeeze into their dress or their trousers, say it's all the fault of the cleaners, who must have shrunk the garment the last time it was dry-cleaned.

You can't go through life blaming the cleaners when you put on some weight. You eventually have to face up to the sad truth: You have been eating too much. The answer is, just eat less—cut out in-between meals completely and eat smaller portions at your regular meals. If it makes you feel nobler or better to say you are on "a diet," go ahead. But it really isn't a diet; it is merely a question of beginning a regimen of normal, sensible, regulated eating habits.

It also doesn't hurt you to go without eating anything at all for a short while. In fact, I think doing so gives your system a vacation, and we all know how nice it is to do nothing for a few days. Maybe your digestive system likes a rest, too. Whenever I suggest this to my daughter Phyllis, she says, "Mother, if there is one thing I don't ever want to be, it's hungry." So she won't do the eat-nothing-at-all bit. I do it occasionally, but never for more than two days at a time. That's long enough, I think, to give my system a bit of a holiday.

Both my daughters, Alice and Phyllis, are bigger than I am, but so is everybody else. It seems to me that the world is full of bigger people today—look at the pro basketball players—and I imagine that's attributable, at least partially, to good eating habits for our children. Plus, of course, the fact that we are giving our youngsters all those vitamins when they are just toddlers. So my daughters grew up bigger boned, bigger footed, stronger and taller and heavier than I am. But neither has a serious weight problem, although Alice, who lives in New Orleans and is a master (or mistress) of that great Cajun cooking, has to watch her weight very closely.

Phil is always fighting to lose a few pounds. Strangely, he has never been a big eater, but still he has that tendency to put on weight at the drop of a snack. In fact, he is an inveterate snacker, and I must tell you what his favorite snack is, although when I do it may turn you off eating entirely for a month. My dear husband loves to fix himself a sandwich composed of crisp bacon, a heavy dose of peanut butter, and several thin slices of raw onion. "Honey," he says, licking his lips, "there is nothing in the world like a bacon, peanut butter, and onion sandwich." Then, at dinnertime, he'll tell me how hungry he is, how he hasn't eaten a thing all day—and the kitchen is full of the remnants of that sandwich-making affair.

Phil is an extremely good cook, however. His corn bread, which he learned to make back home in Indiana, is famous in the musical circles in which he traveled. And I must say it is practically irresistible. He's taught his daughters how to make it, but not me. He says it's one thing he doesn't want me to know. But Alice and Phyllis both make it now, to the delight of their families and friends, who keep begging for the recipe. It is going to stay in the family, though, at least for the time being.

One of Phyllis's best girl friends really needs the recipe for Phil's corn bread, or for something at any rate. She is typical of a lot of American girls who, for one reason or another, have never bothered to learn how to cook much of anything. So this gal, whenever she has a date over for dinner, always serves the same thing: French fries and garlic toast, the only things she knows how to make.

There are some old wives' tales in the area of food that I believe can cause a lot of harm.

One is the widely held notion that your body knows best, so whenever you feel a pang of hunger, it is your body telling you that it needs some nourishment. So, the old wives say, when you are hungry, you have to eat something. That's the rationalization, of course, for nonstop snacking. And non-stop snacking leads, inevitably, to nonstop weight gaining. So when you feel that pang of hunger, ignore it. It isn't your body telling you it needs food, it is your evil self telling you it wants a snack.

As a matter of fact, I find I enjoy the feeling of being slightly hungry. I never want to be really hungry, like those tragic people in Ethiopia and other parts of Africa, so maybe I am being insensitive when I say I enjoy being slightly hungry. But it is true. I know I feel much better being slightly hungry than being slightly overstuffed.

Another old wives' tale that I will gladly debunk is the one that goes, You really should have a little extra weight on you in case, God forbid, you come down with a dread disease. If you are too thin, just skin and bones, they say, you'll go like that, but if you have a few extra pounds, you can fight it off. That's another rationalization for eating more than you should. I don't know if there is any scientific merit to the argument that you can fight disease better with that added weight, but I do know that medical researchers agree that too much added weight can actually cause diseases—high blood pressure, strokes, circulatory problems.

So if I must err in one direction or the other, I would much rather be a little too thin than a little too heavy. It seems to me the safer course. I'm not exactly thin, but I think I'm more thin than I am fat. I was thinner a few years ago, but that was too thin. My face showed it, so I put on a few pounds, my face filled out, and now, I believe, I am right about where I should be in the weight department.

There is one restaurant near my home where I love to go with friends for lunch, or occasionally with Phil for dinner. And one of the specialties of this restaurant is its assortment of rich, gloppy desserts. The waiters and waitresses parade them by, proudly, on their trays. And I watch them go past, and I ooh and aah like all the rest of the patrons. But that's all I do—ooh and aah and watch them go past. I never order one. For me, just looking is pleasure enough. I get the same joy out of looking at a rich dessert as I do out of going to an art gallery and looking at a glorious painting. I don't have to own the painting to experience its beauty, and I don't have to eat that dessert to enjoy it. I don't want to put all that sugar, all those calories, all that valueless material, inside me.

Look but don't touch.

Of course, we are living in a magnificent age for eaters. Science and food processors have combined to create food that is much less harmful than in bygone days. There are sugarless sweeteners, saltless seasonings, oils without cholesterol, ice cream without fat, and on and on. So if you must have desserts and other ordinarily unhealthy items in your daily diet, at least insist they are made from these newly created safer ingredients.

You can't make sure of that when you are dining out, of course, but you can when you are in your own home, and preparing the food yourself. Be sure, when you buy something at the supermarket, to read the label and check the ingredients. (Of course, some manufacturers are so sneaky they print that list of ingredients in such small type it is impossible to read. I know one lady who always goes shopping with a magnifying glass, so she can read the list of ingredients no matter how small the print is.)

Get to know what ingredients you want to avoid. Check with your doctor about that. He or she will be glad to tell you the things you should shun in your state of health. And you will find that most supermarkets nowadays have aisles for "health foods." I find that the canned and packaged foods in those aisles are just as tasty as their counterparts in the rest of the store, and much healthier.

You can always find something that is just as delicious as a food you're not supposed to eat. When I feel the urge for ice cream, for example, I will buy myself some frozen yogurt. The taste is marvelous, and frozen yogurt is full of calcium and has nowhere near the fat, sugar, and calories of ice cream.

Eating in restaurants can be difficult, because most of them naturally try to create dishes that taste fabulous, and that often means fattening and unhealthy sauces and gravies. Besides, you can never be sure what they use in preparing their creations. I try to order something simple—again, pasta is frequently my choice—and often ask them to hold the sauce or at least serve it on the side.

I have seen many people bring food to restaurants with them. I believe it was Zsa Zsa Gabor who would often bring a bunch of grapes to a restaurant and ask the maître d' to serve them as her dinner. And that would be all she would eat.

To sum it all up, one of the main factors contributing to Growing Older but Staying Young is your diet. And my secret weapon is to leave the table wanting more. Eat your normal diet, a balanced diet if you possibly can, but eat a little less of it.

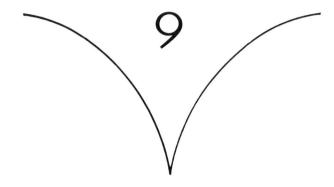

9

This chapter could consist of only four words:

Try not to smoke!

But you would feel cheated if you picked up a book and there was a chapter in it with only four words—I know I would—so I will add a few more.

When boys and girls of my generation were growing up, it seemed the height of maturity and sophistication to smoke a cigarette. It was so elegant, so classy! What we didn't know at the time was that it was also so deadly. Nobody told us that cigarettes were harmful to our health, mostly because scientists had yet to prove that link. They may have suspected there was a cause and effect between cigarette smoking and certain diseases, but they hadn't proved it. And scientists are understandably reluctant to make an accusation like that unless and until it has been proved absolutely. So the boys and girls of my generation began smoking as soon as we could. We became hooked on tobacco innocently; we never knew it was a death warrant for many of us.

The boys and girls of today have no such excuse. If they are dumb enough to start smoking, they do it with their eyes open. They have heard often enough—in fact, it is printed right on the package—that cigarettes are dangerous. They should know better, and I really have very little sympathy for today's kids if they begin smoking. It is just stupid.

Everybody knows the truth today. The hard, cold facts about the dangers of smoking have been aired on television, written about in newspapers and magazines, shown in movies, talked about by everybody from the surgeon general of the United States to your family doctor. But just in case you have missed it, the facts are that smoking can cause any number of fatal conditions—cancer of the lungs is the most notable, but links have also been shown between smoking and heart disease, smoking and strokes, smoking and emphysema, smoking and diseases of the cardiovascular system.

Obviously, not every smoker will be affected by these potential dangers. That is the tragedy, because everybody has an Uncle Harry or an Aunt Jenny who smoked a pack of cigarettes a day and lived to be ninety-three. But Uncle Harry and Aunt Jenny just happened to be lucky. The fact that somebody else smoked and survived doesn't mean you will have the same good fortune.

If you have ever seen somebody dying from lung cancer, you would never risk it. It is a terrible, painful, lingering way to go. If you have ever seen someone suffering from emphysema, wheezing with every agonizing breath, having to tote around his own portable oxygen tank, you would never risk it. If you have ever seen a person with a heart weakened by arteries clogged because of smoking, a person who must rest after every step he or she takes, you would never risk it.

But my generation didn't know about all that. We saw older people smoking and thought, How grand that looks, how utterly sophisticated! So we began smoking. I think I must have sneaked my first cigarette on the fire escape when I was twelve or thirteen. But I was luckier than most, in that I never got really hooked on cigarettes. I just didn't like the taste that much, happily. So, although I would smoke occasionally, and I had to smoke for certain movie roles, I was never a heavy smoker. I never smoked when I was working—unless the part called for it—because smoking seems to affect my sense of balance a bit. So if I had to do a song or a dance number, I would never touch a cigarette, for fear I would fall on my face.

When the news broke about how bad cigarettes were for your health, therefore, I was not as terrified as some. I knew I had never smoked to the point where I had imperiled my health.

The good news is that the harm smoking does to your system is not irreversible. Your lungs, for example, will return to normal—provided, of course, that they are not so far gone that it is too late—in anywhere from six months to two years. Scientists are still debating how long it takes, but they are agreed that it can and does happen.

So it certainly pays to quit. I realize that that is easier said than done, however. Although I have never been through it myself, I know enough people who have tried to quit smoking to understand that it is a pretty tough thing to do. In fact, I knew somebody who was addicted to everything—cocaine, hashish, marijuana, even opium—and he told me that the nicotine habit was the hardest of all to kick. But, obviously, it can be done. Millions of people have done it, so you can do it, too.

You can go to one of the stop smoking clinics. You can buy any of the gimmicks designed to help you stop. You can get yourself hypnotized, or acupunctured, or patterned, or whatever. But the secret of stopping smoking is, first, to convince yourself that it is something you must do. You have to really want to quit before you will quit. And when you have reached that absolute, firm, irrevocable decision, the rest is all downhill. Then it doesn't matter what you use as a crutch—a course or chewing gum or hypnotism or what— you *will* quit.

Phil quit smoking recently, after sixty years or so of heavy smoking. As a matter of fact, one of his biggest hit songs and recordings was called "Smoke! Smoke! Smoke! That Cigarette." Once, when I was talking to a group of young elders and telling them to try to stop smoking, one man got up and said, "How come you talk about not smoking and your own husband's biggest hit was 'Smoke! Smoke! Smoke! That Cigarette'?"

Phil tried to quit innumerable times before he finally succeeded. It took him so long because he simply had not yet reached that point of mental readiness where he could quit. He had not yet decided that he really wanted to quit. So he could quit for a while, but after a week or so I'd see him smoking again, just as he always had. And he had trouble with his breathing, so he is one of those people who certainly should have stopped. He finally quit, when he was mentally ready.

Betty Grable was another like Phil. Poor Betty, God bless her, wouldn't quit. She knew she should, but she went right on smoking, cigarette after cigarette, month after month, year after year. I tried to talk to her, but she wouldn't—or couldn't—listen. So she smoked until the end. It killed her.

From my experiences with both Betty and Phil, I learned that nobody can talk a smoker into quitting. It's a personal decision, and it must be reached by the smoker himself or herself. Nobody else can do much more than have a very slight influence.

And that is why, these days, I never come right out and

say, "Don't smoke." You will have noted that right at the beginning of this chapter I didn't say, "Don't smoke." I said, "Try not to smoke." There is a big difference. You have to want to stop in order to try not to smoke. And if you try, you can succeed. It is well worth the effort. Your life may depend on it.

And, speaking of things your life may depend on, I must mention drugs here. I am not talking about the drugs your doctor may prescribe, but the drugs people take for kicks—marijuana, cocaine, crack, and all the other substances that people can become addicted to. I want to add my one small voice to the growing chorus of people telling you: DON'T! They can kill you. And if they don't actually cause your death they can ruin your life, your marriage, your self-respect, your financial condition, everything.

Alcohol is bad, too, in heavy doses, and if abused it can be just as ruinous as hard drugs.

So, if Growing Older but Staying Young is your goal, then stopping smoking, never using drugs, and drinking only in moderation should be an integral part of it all.

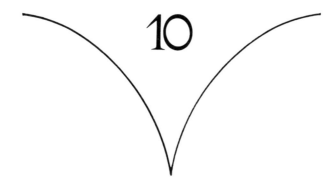

10

Taking care of your body, through exercise and proper eating habits, is important. But it is only half the battle of Growing Older but Staying Young. You also have your mind and your soul to consider. They can get old and rot away, too, if you don't make an effort to keep them young and sprightly.

In our earlier years staying mentally alert and involved and active was never a problem. We all had so much to keep us busy. With some of us, it was our careers. With others, it was managing a home and raising children. And, for many, it was a bit of both. Thus, the problem was never what to do with our time, but rather how to squeeze everything we wanted to do into an already overstuffed day. There just were never enough hours in the day to do everything we really wanted to do.

But now, in our young-elder years, we have the time to do anything we want to do. In fact, for many of us, the problem has become a very serious one: what to do with all those hours in the day. Time, for some, hangs heavy on the hands.

That can be a critical situation. Boredom is an enemy to be battled strenuously. Boredom can erode the mind and the spirit, and cause us to wither away. There is no doubt but that a correlation exists between our physical health and our mental state, that if we are bored and unhappy, our health can suffer. Nature, they say, abhors a vacuum, and boredom is a mental and spiritual vacuum.

So we all have to make a conscious effort to keep ourselves busy, active, involved, up and doing. We cannot sit around, twiddling our thumbs and staring into space. We cannot vegetate. We must exercise our minds as we exercise our bodies.

Even when we were at the studio, pursuing our Hollywood careers, many of us actors felt a need to do something else. We were protected and coddled so much. Our every wish was catered to by studio employees. We didn't have to lift a finger, except to do our jobs in front of the camera. That, in itself, was a little bit oppressive, and there were some stars, I remember, who made a point of finding something, anything, to keep themselves from going stir-crazy.

I remember Joan Bennett as one of those. That beautiful girl kept herself busy by cleaning. Now that may not sound like much to you, but if everything is done for you, then the chance to do a spot of dusting is exciting. Joan would put on an apron and dust her house, even though there were plenty of servants around to do that. And she would vacuum her rugs and carpets. And she would straighten up and scrub the bathrooms and the kitchen. Maybe she was a little obsessive about it, but she once told me that cleaning house was her way of maintaining her sanity in an otherwise basically unreal existence. I can understand that now, although at the time I thought she was a little odd. She simply had to keep busy, keep mentally alert, and acting alone did not satisfy that need in her. So that constant cleaning was her way of staying busy.

I never had any problem staying active during those years. Perhaps it was because, unlike Joan, who was strictly a dramatic actress, I was also a singer and a dancer. For me, there was always a constant round of rehearsals for those musical numbers. Then, after I quit Hollywood, I was busy learning to run a home, taking care of two active little girls and an active and demanding husband. Plus, for quite a few years, I was very busy doing radio and television. So I never had to give a thought to the question of finding something to keep myself active and involved. My problem still was trying to find enough hours in the day to squeeze in all the things I wanted to do.

It was only later, when Alice and Phyllis had grown up and left home, and I wasn't doing so much radio and television anymore, that I had to sit myself down and have a long talk with myself about how I was going to fill up my days. I knew I would spend a lot of time on physical things—my walking and swimming and such—but I also had to stay active for my mind's sake. I just couldn't spend the rest of my life walking and swimming. I had to do something that involved my brain cells. They had to stay functioning, too, or else they would wither on the vine.

There are, fortunately, many things we can do as we reach these young-elder years. There is no law that compels us to sit on our front porches and watch the world go by.

For one thing, the notion that people have to retire when they reach their sixty-fifth birthday is, happily, becoming a thing of the past. Nowadays we know that we can work well beyond that. Sixty-five is still young. Most of us have many productive years left after that. We have all heard of the men and women who have gone on to do marvelous things in their late sixties, their seventies, and even into their eighties and nineties. So, more and more, businesses and industries have abandoned the sixty-five-year-old compulsory retirement rule.

But there are many others who elect to retire at sixty-five and some who even choose early retirement. To them, the idea of a life without having to go to work every day is very appealing. So they quit, take their pensions, apply for their Social Security retirement benefits, and figure they will sit back and do nothing the rest of their lives.

All too often, that period—"the rest of their lives"— becomes short and not so sweet. Total inactivity is dangerous to our health, and many of those retirees wind up dying, a death hastened by the boredom of their totally inactive existences.

So if you can keep working, do so. Maybe your employer will agree, as more and more of them are doing, to allow you to continue to work on a part-time basis. If you are in the white-collar end of the business, perhaps you could continue on as a consultant. A veteran employee staying on the payroll as a consultant makes a lot of sense for everybody—the company has the benefit of the employee's many years of experience, and the employee keeps busy, although in a limited way, allowing him or her plenty of time for relaxation and leisure, too. Even for those men and women who are part of the blue-collar work force, some companies have begun to permit retirement, along with part-time work as instructors of new employees. Expertise in handling machinery or whatever is valuable.

So as your retirement approaches, see if there is some way your company can extend your employment on a part-time basis. You could either continue doing your old job with reduced hours (and a reduced salary, naturally) or just come in for a few hours a week to help teach the new employees.

Either way it gives you something to do, just enough so your mind stays active. And you still wind up with plenty of time for hunting or fishing or golf or bridge playing or whatever it is you want to do with those leisure hours.

If your company can't see their way clear to make such an arrangement, perhaps one of their competitors can. After all, they may have a more enlightened management, which recognizes the potential worth of all your years of experience. Or try a company in some other field. More and more companies in more and more industries today are using part-time workers, especially retirees.

But there are still many thousands of people who want to retire and never lift a finger again. To them, the idea of having to go to work, even on a part-time basis, is for the birds. They are the ones this chapter is aimed at particularly. They are the ones who could be in for a peck of trouble coping with total inactivity. No matter how attractive that concept may appear, it is very perilous to your health.

The first thing I did, when I decided I had to get out and be doing something, was to go to the Eisenhower Medical Center, a marvelous hospital complex in Rancho Mirage, not far from where I live, and ask if there was something I could do.

There was. Hospitals are always delighted to have volunteers. You work a few hours a week, just helping with the patients. Nothing that requires training or experience or any particular skill, just being friendly and helpful. I pushed around a little cart with books and magazines mostly. I would go into the rooms and ask if the patients wanted anything to read, and help them select books or magazines they might like. And while I was there, I would chat with the patients, try to brighten up their days.

I don't know if it brightened up their days very much, but it sure brightened mine. It gave my life a purpose. I know that on the days I was scheduled to work at the hospital, I woke up and bounced out of bed. I had something useful to do! For someone who has spent her lifetime working and then suddenly finds herself at loose ends, it is joyous once again to face a day that has meaning. I am sure the patients I worked with would have survived just as well had I not been there, but I like to think I was helping in some small way.

So for several years I volunteered at the hospital a couple of days every week. For a while I was also working at another of the hospitals in the Coachella Valley—the Desert Hospital in Palm Springs—so I wound up working three and sometimes four days a week. Just a few hours each day, nothing that was overpowering, but enough to keep my mind from rusting away, and to give my life some meaning.

Then they asked me if I could help raise some money for the hospital. I tried, but I wasn't very good at that. I was much better at pushing the cart with books and magazines. I found I just couldn't ask people for money. It was certainly for a worthy cause, and I contributed myself, but I didn't have it in me to go up to somebody and ask for a contribution.

I enjoyed working at the two hospitals and, if I didn't have something to do now—my work for Pfizer Pharmaceuticals—I would certainly be doing that.

If the idea of a hospital turns you off—there are, I realize, many people who are so frightened of hospitals that they wouldn't go near one, even as a volunteer worker—there are other places that would welcome your help as a volunteer. Your local orphanage, or any child-care center, can always use someone who enjoys being around and working with children. You might even find it rewarding to help around a prison, and many such institutions use volunteers in safe areas. Maybe you love animals. If so, your local pound or animal shelter can use an extra hand from time to time.

There is a whole area of volunteer work for men and women willing and able to be docents. If you are not familiar with the word "docent," the dictionary defines it as "a lecturer," but it has come to mean a volunteer guide-lecturer-instructor in a museum or such. Most museums use docents, who can be young elders or people of any age or sex, to take groups of schoolchildren, or interested adults, around. The institutions train them, of course. I know many people who are docents, and the days they work are the high spots of their lives.

In the desert near where I live, there is a miraculous place called The Living Desert, a museum that is totally outdoors. It contains all the flora and fauna of the desert, which is an amazing area, and everything is in its natural habitat. The Living Desert has dozens of docents, guiding tours and talking to the visitors. In your area there are probably four or five places that use docents. It is all volunteer work—museums are generally too strapped for funds to pay anything—but it is helpful work, and, most important to you, it is something that occupies the mind and gives immense personal satisfaction. It can also be a wonderful and valuable learning experience—and you are never too old to learn new things.

Still, that may not appeal to you either. (You are getting very hard to please!) Maybe what you need is a constructive hobby.

At one point, when the volunteer work wasn't enough, I said to Phil, "Honey, I think I'd like to paint."

"Swell," he said. "The house could use a couple of coats."

So much for having an understanding husband. But I went out and bought a set of paints, an easel, the whole works. I had heard about a lot of amateurs painting, and every year there was a show in Palm Springs, where people bought paintings from amateur celebrity painters and the profits went to Barbara Sinatra's work with abused children. So I felt maybe I could paint something and next year somebody might want to buy it, and that would help another worthy cause.

So I started to paint. No lessons, but with oil paints you can blunder ahead on your own. Of course, I probably would have done a lot better had I had a lesson or two, but I was too impatient to get to it. Using oils, you can just cover up your mistakes and nobody is the wiser. For example, in one of my first efforts, I decided to paint a group of boys and girls. They were so ugly I couldn't stand them. So I put hair on all their faces, and, presto, the painting showed the backs of their heads. A very successful painting, if you like to see a bunch of backs of heads.

A Grandma Moses I wasn't. But I had fun. And I found that I could start painting at nine o'clock in the morning and turn around and it was four in the afternoon. Seven hours went by like that. I didn't even stop for lunch; it just never occurred to me to stop, or to be hungry. It was, for me, a great way to spend a day.

And I did have the great joy and satisfaction of having one of my paintings bought at the next year's charity auction. It was a painting I had done of a little girl at the beach. To put the icing on my cake of happiness, I later found out that the person who had bought it was Frank Sinatra.

I have mentioned before that one thing I still want to do in my lifetime is learn to play the piano. You are never too old to learn something new. You can always study something. You can go to school; most colleges and some high schools have extension courses, and they offer everything from languages to bonsai. Whatever interests you, you can probably find a course on it offered at some nearby college or high school. Or you can teach yourself. Your bookstore is chock-full of books (and these days videos) that can give you the rudiments of some new knowledge—carving birds, speaking basic Spanish, learning about astronomy, improving your golf swing, playing the guitar, cooking, whatever.

I know it is that notion of someday learning how to play the piano that still hangs over my head. When I was a little girl back in New York, my poor mother worked her fingers to the bone to pay for piano lessons for me. Then, of course, I was too busy playing outside with the other kids to bother practicing, so I remember nothing from those few lessons. Like so many of us, I regret that folly of my youth. But I realize it's not too late. All I have to do is want to do it badly enough, and I will. And one of these days—

It's not too late for me, although I know I probably will never get to Carnegie Hall. (I already played Carnegie Hall! In fact, I played it twice—in *Alexander's Ragtime Band* I sang there, and then for the gala celebration of the birthday of my friend Hildegarde I was given the honor of bringing her birthday cake out to her on the stage of that venerable hall.)

I believe every one of us has lived for years with a secret, or perhaps not-so-secret, yearning to do something other than what we have been doing all our lives. Now is the time to do it. Besides my painting and the old story of wanting to learn how to play the piano, I have always wanted to be able to spend more time doing needlepoint, which I love, and reading, which I love, and cooking, which I love (at least I love it now that I don't have to do it all the time).

I like to do needlepoint that I then turn into pillows, or sometimes use in other ways around the house.

I am a great reader. I must confess that I buy all the new novels, but my taste is broad—I enjoy reading the autobiographies and biographies of people I admire, and I am fascinated by history.

I also like to do crossword puzzles. Certainly a crossword puzzle is a great exercise for the brain. So I love to pick up a challenging one and see if I can finish it—without having to consult a dictionary or a smart friend.

The thing is, basically, to keep yourself active. I think many of us who came from poor backgrounds, such as I did, had the role models of our mothers and/or grandmothers as shining examples of active, involved women.

My father, who was a New York city policeman, worked hard. But in those days New York cops made very little money—unless they were on the take, and my dad was one of the honest policemen. I never talked to him about that, but I imagine he simply felt (as most policemen do) that his job was to uphold the law, not break it, so if he ever had any opportunities to take bribes, he didn't.

That meant, of course, that we had to scratch to survive. With my grandmother living with us, and me and my two brothers to feed and clothe, it was just too much. So my mother had to go to work. My darling grandmother practically raised me, because my mother was out working all through my childhood. Mom worked for a long time for the Coty perfume people, and she also worked for a chocolate company, which was great for us kids, because she often brought home samples.

So I grew up with the notion that it is very normal for women to work. Of course, I did my share as a young girl—I had to make the beds when I came home from school, and I also had to assist my grandmother as she prepared dinner. It was only after all those chores were attended to that I was able to go outside and play—and then I had to come in at a certain time to do my homework and practice my piano (which I didn't do).

Everybody in my house was active and involved, and I was active and involved all through my early and middle years. The problem was never not having anything to do. On the contrary, the problem was always finding the time to do everything I wanted to do.

That is why the idea of doing nothing is totally alien to my nature. I cannot understand those people who sit around on their keisters day after day, doing nothing but staring into space and daydreaming about past glories. A person can get into a lot of trouble—physically as well as mentally—by drowning in the past. That whole attitude of "I remember when" can be a trap from which there is no escape except the grave. That may sound like a harsh judgment, but I am afraid it is true. If a person does nothing but think about what once was, just sitting idly and letting the old days parade across the mind, he or she is on the road to becoming a vegetable.

Maybe the present isn't so hot. Maybe your children are ignoring you and your living conditions leave a lot to be desired, and maybe life used to be a whole bunch better. That's no excuse to wallow in memories. Get out and do something, and you'll find you'll be able to transform this drab present life into a hopeful future. The key is to become active and involved.

With me, there are days when I could easily let myself slide into a pit of depression. I may sound like I'm always up, but the truth is that there are many mornings when I have to struggle to pull myself out of the gloom. So I have little things I do to give myself a new lease on life. It may only be taking myself to the beauty department at Saks and having my face made up. Maybe I'll buy myself a little present—a pair of shoes or a scarf. Or, even more fun, I buy somebody else something. My biggest kick on a rainy, depressing day is to think of somebody I know who is hospitalized and buy that person some flowers or a box of candy or something to brighten his or her day. Making somebody else happy gives you a big lift.

Of course, my everyday routine is something that I can fall back on, because it gives me solace. Swimming seems to eradicate the blues. I know a lot of my neighbors have swimming pools, as I do, but they use them as decorations. Some have even filled them in with dirt and planted flowering shrubs in them. But mine is utilitarian; I swim in it, as I have said, several times every day. Each time I come out of the pool, I am in a better frame of mind than when I went in, to say nothing of the benefit I have given my body.

So whenever I hear even the faintest whisper of feeling

sorry for myself, I try to drown it out by doing something.

Boredom is the enemy of peace of mind.

And activity is the enemy of boredom.

I realize there are many women who have spent their entire lives in the productive but limiting area of home-making. They have raised their children, cooked, done the laundry and the cleaning, chauffeured in the car pools, den-mothered the Boy Scouts, and contributed so much in so many ways. Now, suddenly, they are, say, fifty, and the last of their children have moved away. Maybe to compound the problem their husbands have died. So there they are, wid-owed and virtually alone, and here I come and say they should become active and involved.

"Doing what?" they may ask. "What can I do? I'm not trained to do anything. I can't get a job because I've never worked, so I have no experience. How can I be active and involved when I'm no good for anything?"

In the first place, as I have said, there is volunteer work. It doesn't take any experience to push a cart around the hospital corridors and hand out books and magazines to pa-tients. Helping others is, as I am sure you must realize, a very rewarding experience. You, as a lifetime homemaker, have spent years helping others, so it should be easy to slide into that niche.

But maybe you would like to earn some money, meaning that volunteer work doesn't appeal to you. More and more, enlightened employers are hiring people just like you, teach-ing them simple skills—obviously it is too late for you to become a computer engineer or an architect, but not too late for you to be taught how to run a computer keyboard or how to file. Go to a good employment agency—there are many in the major cities that specialize in finding jobs for people just like you.

There are some jobs available that might be right up your alley. I hate to be on the receiving end of a telephone sales pitch, but most of those doing the pitching are people like you, who can work from their own homes, making calls to a selected list of prospects and earning a commission on anything they happen to sell.

I doubt if you would want to do any factory work, but I'm told that many factories today hire people like you for certain jobs. Not for running heavy machinery, of course, but for the lighter tasks that do not require either great strength or a lot of training.

But I believe far and away the greatest percentage of young elders I know find they enjoy doing something today that they have wanted to do all their yesterdays. All of us, I think, have harbored a dream that says, "Someday, if I ever have the time, I would really like to learn how to make a hooked rug." Or perhaps, "You know, when the kids have gone out on their own, I think I would love to try to write a novel." Whatever it is, this is your chance to do it. There never will be another chance. It is now or never.

Besides, it is good for you. So you are killing two birds with one dream when you decide to activate that long-standing fantasy.

Go for it.

If you think it sounds silly, don't tell anybody. Jean Auel decided she wanted to write some books about prehistoric times, but she felt people would laugh at her if she said that was what she was doing. So she didn't tell a soul, and it wasn't until *The Clan of the Cave Bear* was published and became a big hit that anybody knew that that nice Mrs. Auel down the street had written a book. Grandma Moses began daubing away with her paintbrush when she was well into her seventies, but none of her friends and neighbors and many in her family were unaware that that was what she was doing until after she was "discovered" and began selling her paintings for astronomical sums of money.

Now obviously we can't all become as successful as Jean

Auel or Grandma Moses. But I would wager that the important thing to both those women was not so much the success as the act of doing something itself. Sure the success was pleasant, but it was, I believe, the icing on the cake; the cake itself would have been sufficient.

As a matter of fact, this thing that you have long wanted to do need not be particularly creative. Maybe you have had the burning desire to go out to the track and bet on the horses. I do not want to go on the record as encouraging gambling, but if that is your heart's desire, do it.

For example, Cary Grant went to Santa Anita or Hollywood Park almost every day, and he bet on every race. He only bet the minimum—two dollars—and if he could find somebody who wanted to bet on the same horse he did, he would suggest they split the cost of a two-dollar ticket. So very often his total wager was one dollar. You can do something like that, if you do it prudently.

The whole point of this chapter can be summed up in a few simple words:

Get active. Get involved. Do something.

It is important for the sake of your mind, your soul. It is a vital part of the entire concept of Growing Older but Staying Young.

I was sort of at loose ends some years ago, when I happened to be invited to be a guest on her show by my old friend Mary Martin. She has a home near me in Rancho Mirage, and we had become quite close over the years. She was cohosting a PBS program aimed at young elders, so she frequently had guests on of our mutual generation. I was very happy to be on the show, which came from San Francisco. We had a lovely time. During the course of our conversation, Mary asked me what I was doing, and I had to confess I was doing nothing.

"Just swimming and walking," I said.

She shook her head. "You should be doing more," she

said. "You have to keep yourself active and involved."

Her words were echoing in my mind when, by coincidence, I received a letter from the Pfizer people a few days later. They asked me to work for them. They said I could travel, on their behalf, to places where there were meetings of young elders and talk to them about myself, answer some questions, give them some advice about Growing Older but Staying Young—although they hadn't coined that phrase. I called Mary and told her about the offer. She said, "Go for it, Alice," and I went for it.

Now, perhaps a dozen times a year, I do travel for Pfizer; I meet so many wonderful people. It is just enough so I keep myself occupied, but not so much that it is exhausting.

So I am a working woman again, and I love it. I am practicing what I preach: Stay active and involved!

Thank you, Mary Martin.

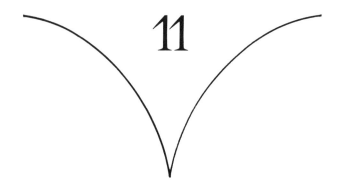

11

When I was a little girl I would have had to be practically on death's door before my family would have called a doctor. And since I was a very healthy child, and never even came close to death's door, I don't remember ever seeing a doctor. The home remedies of my Irish grandmother saw me through whatever crises I may have confronted. It wasn't that my folks were antidoctor particularly. It was just that, in those pre–health insurance days and given their income, a doctor was a luxury they could not afford. Doctors and hospitals were for the rich, or the dying.

My attitude, and I think the attitude of the entire public, toward the medical profession has changed radically. Perhaps it was the influence of the doctor shows on television, such as "Dr. Kildare" or "Ben Casey" or "Marcus Welby, M.D." Or maybe it was the advent of medical insurance programs, or the government-supported programs such as Medicare, which have reduced the cost to the patient of seeing a doctor or going to a hospital. Or, probably, it is a combination of both these factors, plus the realization that it makes sense to see a doctor.

In any event, the point of this chapter is to tell you that, if you want to practice Growing Older but Staying Young, one thing you have to do is see your doctor regularly.

We all have read statistics that tell us our life expectancy is lengthening. When I was a girl, it was a rare thing for someone to live into his or her eighties. Today it is common. My own theory about that—there are other contributing factors, of course—is that nowadays we do consult doctors more frequently. It stands to reason that if you have an annual checkup, and the doctor detects a condition that can be controlled or totally eradicated, you will live longer than if you had not seen the doctor and that condition had been allowed to increase unchecked.

Most diseases—even cancer—can be beaten if they are discovered early enough. And the only way to discover them early is to have that annual checkup.

In my case, the high blood pressure I have was first found by my doctor during one of those routine checkups. High blood pressure, as I will discuss in detail in the next chapter, is one of those insidious things that can occur without producing any symptoms you can feel. So the only way to find out if you have it is to have your doctor test your blood pressure. My doctor immediately prescribed medication that now keeps my blood pressure within safe limits. But had I not gone to see him for that checkup, and not found out what was going on inside my body, I probably would have been dead long before this.

Actually, I try to have a checkup now every six months. And I go to my doctor more often if I feel something is wrong. I think I owe it to myself to let him tell me if whatever is bothering me is serious or not. I do not think I am a hypo-chondriac, or even close to being one. I simply believe my health is a very important thing. Going to the doctor only takes a few minutes, and it puts my mind at ease. And some-times it puts my body at ease, too.

The cost of seeing a doctor is a deterrent, of course. But the various medical plans and insurance programs are bring-ing that cost down somewhat. I grant you that going to see a doctor frequently is an expensive business. Yet I feel strongly that, whatever it costs, it is worth every penny. Can you put a price on your life? What is the value of time? How much are a few more years, to see your grandchildren grow up, worth to you?

I truly believe that my own life has been extended be-cause I have made conscientious visits to my doctor. He found my high blood pressure and gave me the medicine to keep that controlled. When I went to him about my arthritis, he told me what I could do to lessen the pain, so my life is not as difficult to bear as it might have been. Time after time he has helped me with some things that are life threatening and other things that make life harder to take.

But perhaps you don't have a doctor. How do you go about getting a doctor who is qualified and who you like?

You should shop for a doctor, just as you would shop for an auto mechanic or a plumber. Begin by asking friends or relatives for a recommendation. Do they have a doctor they trust, someone they have a rapport with? Go to see him (or her, because more and more women are becoming doctors these days). Talk to the doctor, explain that you are looking for a personal physician. Ask about his or her training, about charges, just talk. See if you seem to feel an empathy with the doctor. Most physicians welcome this kind of preliminary conversation. If, however, the one you are meeting gives you the brush-off, cross him or her off your list.

If you cannot get a recommendation from friends or

relatives, call your local medical association. It will probably be listed in your telephone book under the name of your county—where I live, in Riverside County, it is listed as Riverside County Medical Association. Call and ask them to recommend a doctor. The practice is generally to give you three names, not just one. Call all three, and see each of them. Again, try to find one with whom you have a rapport.

This business of establishing a rapport may sound like a frivolous waste of time and energy. It's not. When you are entrusting your life to somebody, that somebody must be a person you trust implicitly. I don't mean that you have to find a doctor who will become your best friend. In fact, there is no law that says you even have to like him or her particularly. But you have to believe in your doctor, believe in his ability, believe that he truly cares about you and your well-being. For instance, some doctors are gruff and terse, with a bedside manner like Godzilla. But somehow you are sure that they know their business, and you just feel safe and secure with them looking after you.

Once you have found a doctor you feel comfortable with, have him or her give you a thorough physical examination. This will be the starting point, the basis of reference. It is best for you to first meet your doctor, and be examined, when you are fine and healthy. That way the doctor knows how your body tests when there is nothing wrong with it.

Being human beings, however, we will probably seek out a doctor when we are sick. So that first physical will most likely occur when you have a bad cold or inflammation of the elbow or something. Still, try to go back to the doctor after you are over the cold or the elbow swelling has gone down. Let him or her give you a complete battery of tests—test your blood and urine, x-ray your chest and do an EKG to see how your heart functions. That way the doctor will have a record of how your body tests when all systems are go.

Then, even before you leave the office, make an appointment for your next examination. It will probably be a year later. However, if there is something the doctor wants to keep an eye on, it will be sooner—six months, or maybe even only three months. Whatever it is, keep that date. Write it down in your appointment book, and be there on time.

Most Americans take better care of their cars than they do of their own bodies. When they buy a new car, they carefully read the owner's manual that comes with it, and if they are told to bring the car in every 7,500 miles for a checkup, they bring it in on the dot. Not 7,499 or 7,501 miles, but exactly at 7,500. But they diddle and dawdle and procrastinate when it comes to seeing their doctors. If their doctors say they want to see them again in a year, they wait a year and three months, or until they have strep throat, whichever comes later.

You can always get a new car. You can never get a new body. So it seems to me we should take better care of ourselves than of our cars. So make a point of having that checkup whenever your doctor says you should—annually, semiannually, or every three months.

That, however, is only half the battle. The other half is to do what the doctor tells you.

Let's assume that your doctor, after the examination, finds there's a little too much sugar in your blood. He says it is nothing to worry about, at the moment, "It's just something I want to keep an eye on." Then he gives you a prescription. It is for a drug that will help lower the blood sugar. He says that if it gets too high, it's a sign of diabetes and eventually, if it continues to climb, you might have to go on insulin. "Meanwhile," he says, "get this prescription filled, take these pills, and that ought to do the trick."

So you go home and figure, well, the doctor said it wasn't anything to worry about. So you won't worry about it. You stick the prescription in the kitchen drawer—the one with all the elastic bands and buttons and old Popsicle sticks—and promptly forget about it. And in a few years you've got diabetes and, to save your life, you have to give yourself an insulin shot every day. Perhaps if you had filled that prescription and begun taking that medicine, you could have thwarted the diabetes and never had to have an insulin shot.

The point is that the doctor doesn't give you a prescription for the fun of it. Nor does he make a dime off of the medicine he is suggesting you buy and take. He is merely telling you that you had better do something now if you don't want bigger trouble later. It's the old "ounce of prevention" routine.

So not only should you see your doctor regularly but you should do what he or she says. Get the prescription filled first, then take your medicine on the schedule suggested, as well as doing whatever else the doctor may tell you to do. It may be changing your diet or beginning a program of exercise or stopping smoking or any of a number of possibilities. Do what the doctor tells you. After all, you have paid him or her a lot of money to help you. It just doesn't make sense to pay out all that hard-earned cash and then ignore your doctor's advice.

To go back to the analogy with your car, if your mechanic said that the reason your car is wheezing is that it needs a new air filter, you wouldn't say, "Gee, thanks," and then go home and forget it. You'd get a new air filter, right now. Why, then, do so many of us choose to ignore what our doctors tell us to do? It's really very foolish, but I know a great many people do just that.

Get your prescriptions filled, and then take the medicines as directed. Those directions are very important, too. If the label on the bottle says, "Take with meals," then by all means take the pill with meals. The reason is that if you take that particular pill on an empty stomach, you probably will upset your digestive system. And if the label says, "Take before bedtime," take it at bedtime. Again, there is a reason—

this particular medicine probably has a tendency to make you drowsy, so it might be dangerous to take in midafternoon, say, when you could nod off while you were driving.

While on the subject of pills, I do want to caution you about swapping pills with other people, or borrowing pills from them. It is a very foolish thing to do. I know it is so common for one person to say, "I have an awful pain in my lower back, right there," and a good friend to say, "I had the same thing and the doctor gave me these pills and I took two and my pain went away, like that. Here, let me give you a couple of them." Or, a person may say to a friend, "Gee, I forgot to bring my high blood pressure pills to the poker game. Can I borrow one of yours?"

Very dumb—dangerously dumb.

The doctor prescribed those pills for that individual, knowing that person's tolerances and conditions. But the pill borrower is an entirely different person and may have different tolerances and conditions. What is good for you may not necessarily be good for me. In fact, it might do me serious harm. Mrs. X's pills, which work wonders for her, could produce a terribly bad reaction in Mrs. Y.

Besides, you can't be sure that the good-hearted person who is lending you those pills has grabbed the right bottle. Just possibly instead of the pills that helped her lower back problem, she grabbed the pills she got last year for her kidney discomfort. So you may be swallowing something that not only is not designed for your problem but could be very bad for your system.

Never borrow pills from anybody else, no matter how tempting the offer may be. And it follows, never be a lender either.

Speaking of pills, what about vitamins? And what about other fad things we can buy across the counter? What about all those remedies we hear touted on TV or see advertised in the slick magazines?

Don't take anything unless you talk it over with your doctor first. Or at least a pharmacist you feel is trustworthy.

It may seem harmless to take a bunch of vitamins. I know a lot of people who bring their pillboxes to the table with them and take six, eight, maybe even a dozen different pills before lunch. They tell you they feel great and it's all because of all the vitamins they take. But my doctor friends tell me that a lot of the vitamins on the market today are placebos at best. Furthermore, you can overload your system if you take too many of certain kinds of vitamins.

I just don't want to take any pill of any sort unless I have to. So, without my doctor's approval, I take zilch. At the moment, I take some vitamin E. My doctor calls that "an all-around good vitamin." When I travel, I take some vitamin C to ward off colds. I used to take an iron supplement, but my doctor told me that once you're past fifty, iron really doesn't help you anymore, so I've stopped taking that.

There are fads involving certain drugs or dietary supplements, as there are fads in every other phase of life. For a time women were taking estrogen as a way of warding off the onset of the years. There was another fad of liquid protein, as a way of staying slim. My doctor told me that both of those things could cause trouble. He actually forbade my taking the estrogen. I was afraid of it, so I never took it.

There are people, I know, who enjoy buying all the latest fad medications and have fun with their little pillboxes with the different colors, to remind them of when to take what. But I'm just the opposite; I take nothing that the doctor hasn't advised me to take. And even when my doctor does advise me to take something, I make a nuisance of myself asking him to tell me the whys and the wherefores of the prescription.

He doesn't mind. That's part of his job. And there are certain things you *should* ask your doctor when he or she prescribes a new medication for you. You have a right to know.

You should ask, first, what is the medication supposed to do for you?

Then you should ask the doctor to spell out, in simple and clear terms, how often you should take it and under what conditions. Should it be taken in the morning? with meals? with a liquid?

Next, of course, ask about any potential side effects the medicine might produce. Are they the kind of side effects that may be severe? If so, should you continue to take the medication or stop if and when those side effects appear? If you stop taking it, will that cause any problem?

Remind the doctor of any other medications you may be taking. He or she probably doesn't need a reminder, because all that information is on your chart, but remind the doctor anyhow. Better to be on the safe side. Some medications interact with others in a harmful way, so ask the doctor if there is any potential problem in adding this new medication to what you are already taking.

Tell him about any allergies you may have. This fact could play a big role in the medication he prescribes for you. If your doctor is unaware of those allergies, he could prescribe something that might be harmful to you.

Then, when you go to your pharmacy to get the new prescription filled, you might continue asking questions, this time of your pharmacist.

Ask if there is a generic alternative to what your doctor prescribed. The generics are less expensive than the brand-name drugs.

Ask, too, about the longevity of the drugs you are buying. Perhaps you only have to take a few of the pills, and you have a right to know if the ones left in the bottle should then be thrown away or can be stored. There are some drugs that not only don't last but turn into harmful substances if kept too long. Also ask the pharmacist (if your new medication is in a capsule) if it can be taken with hot food.

Try, if possible, to match your medication, and the times and method of taking it, to your life-style. The easier it is for you to take, the less chance there will be of your forgetting it. Make it a habit. That word—"habit"—has come to have a bad meaning, and lots of us don't want to get in the habit of doing anything. But if what you are doing is good for you, then the habit, too, is a good one. And if you can get into the habit of taking your pills on a certain schedule, it is very beneficial. First, it makes it hard for you to overlook taking them, and, equally important, your body likes doing things at the same time every day. So it likes knowing that a certain medication will be arriving in the stomach every day at a certain hour. It can object to haphazard medication schedules.

Don't think because your doctor prescribes some drug for you that you are a medical pioneer, or a human guinea pig, or blazing new trails in science. It is common knowledge that the majority of people in the United States who are sixty-five or older take some medication every day.

You are also not all alone out on some limb if your doctor tells you you have one of the chronic illnesses that affect people in this age bracket. Four out of five people who are over sixty-five have at least one of the common chronic illnesses of this age-group—high blood pressure, arthritis, diabetes, or cancer. So you should not be surprised if you hear from your doctor that you have one of these conditions. Actually, you should be expecting it.

But the thing is that now, with all the marvelous advances medicine is making every day, these conditions are generally manageable. In past years if you heard that you had cancer, you would understandably think it was all over. Today, assuming it is diagnosed in time, your chances of living many more years—and quality years, at that—are good.

But you have to work with your doctor. Say, for example,

he tells you you have high blood pressure, as I do. He will start by prescribing a particular drug. He will want to see how it works with you. My doctor friends tell me that no drug yet discovered has no side effects—even aspirin can sometimes affect the digestive system. So the doctor will want you to tell him if the drug he has given you bothers you in any way—does it make you drowsy, does it upset your stomach, does it give you headaches? And he will want to see if the drug is doing the job it is intended for. Is it lowering your blood pressure?

If the side effects are too severe, or if your blood pressure has not gone down as much as he'd hoped, he will change your drug. There were, at last count, thirty-six different drugs designed to control high blood pressure. Your doctor will ask you to try one after another until he finds one that is working without producing side effects that are too severe. Maybe the very first drug he prescribes will be the one that is best for you, but maybe it will take ten or more tries before he settles on the one that is best.

You owe it to yourself to cooperate with him fully as he works to find the drug with the optimum success. He will probably tell you to call him in a few days to report on how you feel. Call him right on schedule and explain, briefly but in sufficient detail, if the drug seems to be having any adverse effect on you. He will want to see you in a few weeks to check your blood pressure. Be sure to show up on time.

"My doctor can't seem to make up his mind what drug he wants me to take," one woman said to me. "He keeps changing my prescription. He's a jerk." No, he isn't the jerk. That woman is the jerk. It wasn't that he couldn't make up his mind, he was just trying to pinpoint the one drug that was the best for her to take.

When your doctor asks you how you feel after you have taken a new medication for a few days, speak up and mention everything, even if it seems insignificant. Maybe it is just a little feeling of fatigue. Or a slight loss of appetite. Or a vague sense of depression. All of those, minor though they may seem, could be side effects of the medication. Maybe another drug could produce good results without any side effects at all. But the doctor will never know about that fatigue, that loss of appetite, that depression, unless you tell him or her.

I know people who begin taking a medication and have some peculiar feeling—such as loss of appetite—and they say, "Well, I guess I'm just getting a little old." They never make the connection between the drug they have started taking and that loss of appetite. It probably isn't aging, it probably is a side effect.

My own doctor has a tough time with me, because medication, by and large, doesn't agree with me. I react badly to most drugs, and that makes it difficult for both of us. My doctor will prescribe something for me, and I'll get queasy and tell him about it, and he'll say, "OK, let's try something else," and he'll write me a prescription for a different drug. Often I will have to try three or four before finding one that helps me without making me feel like I swallowed a crocodile.

What about getting a second opinion? I think that's a good idea if something serious, such as surgery, is involved. For ordinary medical situations, it seems to me to be an unnecessary expense. If you have found a doctor you trust, then trust him. If, however, he suggests an operation to remove your upper liver, I think you should get a second opinion.

Only once in my lifetime have I asked for a second opinion. That time, my doctor advised me to have some nodules removed from my throat. The idea of somebody cutting into my throat didn't fill me with great anticipation, so I had a second opinion. That doctor concurred, so I had it done. I was lucky. They got them out in time—another triumph for early diagnosis—and I walked away without any trauma.

Now I find I'm like President Reagan; we both grow nodules like the farmer in the dell grows radishes. I have to have that part of my anatomy checked a couple of times a year.

Another problem I have is with occasional dizzy spells. One night I sat down to have dinner, admiring the palm trees outside the window. Suddenly the palm trees were revolving, and that's something palm trees do not ordinarily do. I had to lie down.

Another time, in New York, my friend Jewel Baxter and I had gone to see Ruby Keeler in the musical *42nd Street*. (Ruby is a neighbor of mine in California, so I wanted to see her show.) Afterwards, Jewel and I and Patsy Kelly and some others went to get something to eat. I stepped out of the cab and, whammo, that was the end of me. The sidewalk revolved and the street started spinning. I had to grab a lamppost to keep from falling. I know the people who saw me were saying, "Yep, another Hollywood drunk."

They took me back to my hotel, and I couldn't get out of bed for six days. Even when I finally got on the plane to fly home, I was teetering, and I know the other passengers stayed away from me, figuring I was stewed to the gills.

Mamie Eisenhower had the same problem—vertigo. And that's why that poor lady had the reputation of being a drunkard. But I was at quite a few parties where she was also a guest, and I never once saw her drink anything alcoholic except maybe a glass of champagne once in a while. She just had frequent dizzy spells, which make you stagger pretty good.

There isn't much that can be done for that. I've talked to quite a few doctors. It is, they agree, a problem in the inner ear. A little Dramamine—the seasickness preventative—is of some assistance. But really all you can do is wait it out; eventually it goes away by itself.

Still, I mention it to my doctor whenever it happens. It is, after all, a part of my medical profile, and if my doctor is to treat me, I feel he has to know everything about my physical makeup.

There is always something to watch, some minor complaint I have told him about that he is keeping his eye on. He asks me questions, and I try to answer as completely as I can, without taking all day.

You should try to talk to your doctor, as well as listen to him. He cannot help you unless you first explain to him what is bothering you. Sometimes, I realize, that conversational rapport is tough to establish. Some doctors are so rushed, so brusque, that talking to them is like talking to Rambo. But be persistent. I believe ninety-nine doctors out of a hundred really care about you and how you feel. If they seem brusque, it is because they are so pressed for time that they can't dawdle. But don't let your doctor intimidate you. After all, you are paying him or her good money—and plenty of it—so the least your doctor can do is listen to your problem.

On the other hand, there are some people who simply like to hear themselves talk. They are so wrapped up in themselves that they just ramble on and on, and, if nobody stopped them, they could talk endlessly about that pimple on their big toe.

There is a happy medium. If your doctor sees that you are not one of those motor mouths, those ramblers, but simply want to tell him or her, concisely and briefly, about your problem, the doctor will listen with both ears.

One final word of caution about your pills. When you travel, as I do so often in my work for Pfizer, never put your pills in the suitcase you check through. As we all know, the airlines are prone to losing luggage. And, if you are dependent on a particular medication, it could be a disaster, quite possibly life threatening, if your pills are lost with your luggage. I always carry my pills on board with me, in a tote bag or some form of carry-on luggage. This way my pills are with me, even if the luggage is misplaced.

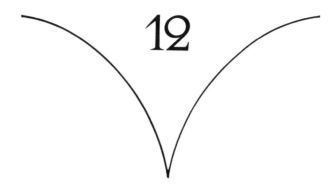

12

The main reason, of course, why you should see your doctor on a regular basis and follow his or her instructions is so you will stay alive for a little longer. The alternative is a bit too final for my taste. And while we are living, we want to feel well. Life itself is fine and dandy, but if the quality of your life is inferior, life loses a great deal of its luster. So you see the doctor and do what he or she suggests to keep yourself going and to feel your best.

When we talk about Growing Older but Staying Young, we are talking about feeling good and looking good. The two are, in my opinion, flip sides of the same coin. No matter how much paint and powder you use, you really cannot look good until and unless you also feel good. Without good health, nothing else really matters. Morale, spirits, mood—call it whatever you choose, it is all the same thing. It is how we feel inside, and if we are bogged down with physical ailments, we feel rotten, and that is immediately reflected in our outward appearance.

The longer we live, the greater our chances of getting something that will hamper our ability to enjoy ourselves, or even something with more dire results.

One of my husband's big hits was a song called "Some Little Bug Is Going to Get You Some Day." The chorus goes:

> Some little bug is gonna get you some day.
> Some little bug is gonna get you some day.
> And then he'll send for his bug friends
> And all your earthly trouble ends,
> Some little bug is gonna get you some day.

The verses elaborate on this theme, detailing how there is danger in everything we eat and drink. One verse, for example, goes like this:

> There are germs of every kind
> In any food that you can find
> Either in your market or on the bill of fare.
> People die from drinking whiskey
> But drinking water's just as risky
> And it's often a bad mistake to breathe the air.

It's a funny song, and it still gets laughs when Phil plays it or sings it. But the underlying message is very serious.

Some little bug will probably get us all someday. And the longer we live, the shorter the odds against us catching something serious. It is virtually inevitable that some catastrophic disease will catch up with every one of us eventually. It's really only a question of what, and when.

In this chapter I want to talk about the most common and most frequent diseases that strike us in our later years. And I want to discuss two very important aspects of those diseases:

1. How to avoid them, if possible

2. How to treat and control them, so you can live with them with as little discomfort as possible

Obviously, there are some things completely beyond our power to avoid. As everyone knows, one of the greatest dangers facing us in our young-elder years is falling and breaking a bone. Bones become more fragile as we get older, and the healing process takes longer. Eventually, total healing becomes almost an impossibility. We must all be careful about falling, but that's about the extent of the preventive measures we can take. No words of mine will be of any help if you trip, fall, and break your hip. Nor can I write anything that will be of any value if you get bitten by a rabid pit bull or if you are attacked by a berserk malaria-carrying mosquito. We all take our chances with life, and we all know it can be a chancy business. Life sometimes has a nasty, dirty trick up its quirky sleeve.

What I am talking about here are not those unavoidable surprises but rather some things over which we can, and should, exercise a modicum of control. And the most common diseases affecting us in our later years are things that we can control to some extent, or at least modify.

Those of us who are in, or fast approaching, our young-elder years, must consider ourselves truly fortunate. Medical and scientific advances have given us a fighting chance in combating diseases that a generation ago were crippling, limiting, debilitating, and very often killing:

High blood pressure and the associated heart disease and strokes, for one.

Osteoarthritis for another.

Diabetes for a third.

And cancer.

Within certain limitations, all of these diseases today are controllable. We may not yet know how to conquer them, but we have learned to live with them. And generally we can live with them in relative comfort.

Of course, there are still some conditions science has yet to get a handle on. Alzheimer's disease, for one. But it is almost certain that someday scientists will conquer it too. They will find either a way to prevent it or a way to cure it, perhaps even both. At the moment, however, medical science cannot prevent the onset of Alzheimer's disease, nor can it cure the disease if it strikes. Let us hope and pray that, very soon, that gap in medicine will be plugged.

But this chapter is about diseases we *can* control.

HIGH BLOOD PRESSURE: High blood pressure, for example. (I seem always to mention that first; perhaps that is because I have it myself.) High blood pressure is an insidious affliction, because it produces no obvious symptoms. People can have high blood pressure, and be slowly dying from its effects, yet feel fine for months, even years. It can be detected only by the sphygmomanometer, which is a word I will never say again. Let's just call it the high blood pressure gauge. It is the device with the rubber sleeve the doctor wraps around your arm, then squeezes with a bulb.

Our grandparents, and even our parents, if they were the victims of hypertension (high blood pressure), were doomed to lead severely restricted lives. It was either that or die at an early age. No work, no physical or mental stress was permitted. But today those of us with high blood pressure have a good shot at leading a normal life, and a long one.

I am no doctor, so I am not going to try to explain what all is going on inside your body to cause your blood pressure to rise dangerously. Anyhow, from what I understand from my doctor friends, there are several sorts of high blood pressure, many possible causes for these different sorts, a lot of ways something can go wrong inside your body to cause the condition to develop.

But this is not a medical textbook, and we are concerned not so much with how these conditions and diseases begin as with what we can do about them. So I am going to talk about three points: high blood pressure is a potentially very serious thing, so you should have your blood pressure checked frequently, because this is a condition that can be controlled.

First, the seriousness of it. That fact that your blood pressure is high is not in itself a threat to life and limb. But the problem is that high blood pressure can lead to, and actually cause, other things, such as heart attacks and strokes.

If high blood pressure is left untreated, the entire cardiovascular system—heart, veins, arteries, all that good stuff—can eventually be damaged beyond easy repair. This doesn't happen overnight. In fact, it takes considerable time. Patients have been known to have high blood pressure for twenty years or more before the condition produces any tangible trouble. But by the time that trouble is recognized, it is usually too late to do much about it. The damage has been done. High blood pressure causes such drastic changes in the body that they are very often fatal. So if you figure, well, maybe I have high blood pressure, but I feel fine so the heck with it, the chances are that someday you will wake up in a hospital ward with a sheet over your face.

No, the time to do something about high blood pressure is as soon as your doctor detects it. Begin treating it *before* there are any symptoms, other than what the doctor reads on that high blood pressure gauge.

In the previous chapter I told you about the importance of seeing your doctor on a regular basis. If you follow this advice, you know that your doctor always takes your blood pressure. It is routine, automatic. The sooner any disease or condition is spotted and diagnosed, the better your chances of beating it. That goes especially for high blood pressure. If the doctor finds it when you are young, when, presumably, it has only recently begun, it can be controlled. Then you can live with it, because it no longer constitutes a serious threat to your well-being.

When the doctor checks your blood pressure, he or she will give you two numbers, for example, "Mr. Brown, your blood pressure is one twenty-five over eighty-five." The first figure—the 125—is called the systolic pressure. That is the measure of the blood as it presses against the walls of your arteries when your heart expels it. Your doctor monitored that pressure when the rubber sleeve wrapped around your arm was pumped full of air, which temporarily prevented the blood from flowing. The second figure—the 85—is called the diastolic pressure. That is the measurement of the pressure on the walls of your arteries between heartbeats. It is, therefore, the more critical figure, since it shows the least amount of pressure your arteries must withstand.

It is impossible for me to tell you what those figures should be in your case, since they vary considerably, depending on factors such as age, sex, weight, heredity, and general state of health. Your doctor will tell you if the figures for you are within a normal range. If they are, you don't have to be concerned. But your doctor may say, "Well, Mr. Brown, it looks like we have a little problem here—your blood pressure is a little too high, and we have to do something about it."

What is fortunate is that, as I mentioned before, there are different drugs designed to lower the blood pressure. Your high blood pressure is never "cured," however. It is merely brought under control. The medication makes it possible for your blood pressure to be reduced to within normal limits. But it is only the medication that is doing this. If you stopped taking your pills for a few days, the pressure would once again shoot up to the danger zone. So you will have to take your medication for the rest of your life. I realize that that is a difficult prospect to grasp, but I believe the alternative is considerably more grim. If you don't take those pills, like clockwork every day for the rest of your life, you will almost surely have a serious problem at some point, such as a heart attack or a stroke. Isn't it far better to swallow a couple of pills a day than to have a heart attack?

My own case has followed the classic scenario. During a semiannual physical checkup some five or six years ago, my doctor took my blood pressure. Then he gave me that routine about "It looks like we have a little problem here." I always get a kick out of the way doctors use that plural pronoun "we." It is somehow comforting to me to realize that my doctor feels that my problem is also his problem. I feel better knowing that I am not alone in my struggle against whatever it is; I have a good, strong ally standing beside me.

Anyhow, this time the problem "we" faced was the fact that my blood pressure was registering too high. I have never been too good about taking pills, but this time the doctor impressed upon me the need to take them regularly. So, since we settled on the best medication for me, I have been taking my pills every single day. And now, whenever my blood pressure is taken, it registers well within normal limits. No problem. So that condition is on hold, and I am fine.

The last time I saw my doctor, and he said, "Well, Alice, your blood pressure couldn't be better," I said, "Doctor, how long do I have to keep taking these pills if my blood pressure couldn't be better?" I knew the answer, of course, but I guess all of us live with the hope that our own cases will be different from everybody else's.

"Don't fool around, Alice," the doctor said. "You've got it controlled, and that's because you take your medication. Don't rock the boat." So I didn't argue. I just had my prescription refilled and realized that taking a couple of pills a day is a small price to pay for continued good health. You just have to get into the habit of doing it at a certain time of day, and make it as routine as brushing your teeth or putting on your wristwatch.

Speaking of daily habits, I remember talking to Mary Ann Mobley, the lovely ex–Miss America who is married to Gary Collins. Mary Ann comes from a family of beauties in Mississippi, and she told me about her grandmother. At the time we talked, her grandmother was in her nineties, still going strong and still beautiful. "My grandmother," Mary Ann said, "drinks a glass of lemon juice and water every morning of her life. She often told me that lemon juice and water is a broom for the body. She would say that it swept out the insides and made everything in your body nice and clean."

So if you find yourself sentenced to a lifetime of taking medication to control hypertension, just accept it, and make that pill taking part of your daily routine. Keep the pills, perhaps, in your medicine chest next to the toothpaste, and take them right after you brush your teeth. Or before. But tie the pill taking to some regular facet of your life; that way it becomes easy to remember.

You'll probably resent it for a while. I know I did. Even though I knew, intellectually, that this was a good thing I was doing, still I resented the idea that I had to take those pills, and would have to take them for the rest of my life. I couldn't help but moan that age-old moan, "Why me?"

Scientists cannot answer that moan. They simply do not know why some people get hypertension and others don't. There is some suspicion that heredity plays a part in the selection process. Other theories are that people who lead particularly stressful lives run a greater risk of having high blood pressure, that a diet heavy in salt can bring it on, that black people are more susceptible than white, and that being overweight is asking for high blood pressure trouble.

One curious statistic relates to age and sex. The incidence of high blood pressure is greater among younger men and among older women. Women under fifty are rarely affected, whereas men in that age-group frequently are. Conversely, over fifty it is women who suffer from high blood pressure more than men. Nobody can explain this odd fact.

You might ask if there isn't perhaps some alternative to pills, some other way to control high blood pressure.

If there is some clear-cut cause of the high blood pressure, there may be an alternative. But only in a few cases. For example, someone who is decidedly overweight may be put on a rigorous diet. The doctor may feel that if that person loses fifty pounds or so, his or her blood pressure will come down.

And some doctors believe strongly in the importance of what we eat in controlling blood pressure. One of the bases of the Pritikin theory is that high blood pressure and other similar conditions can be controlled through monitoring what is eaten. And some of their results have been encouraging. Others are experimenting with programs that combine diet regulation with exercise.

But, by far, most doctors, while encouraging good eating habits and plenty of exercise, also believe very strongly that the best, quickest, and surest way of reducing high blood pressure is through medication. And since this medication, if taken according to your doctor's instructions, cannot possibly harm you, why not take the pills and probably extend your life by a few years?

When I say these drugs cannot possibly harm you, I am assuming that you have told your doctor everything. Before he or she prescribes a medication for you, the doctor must know many things about you. Be frank and honest with him—tell him everything he wants to know—because it is your health and well-being that is at stake.

And, as I said before, the doctor must also know what other drugs, if any, you are presently taking. Drugs, after all, are chemicals, and some chemicals react with each other in ways that could cause problems for your body. Presumably your doctor knows what drugs you are taking—if you have

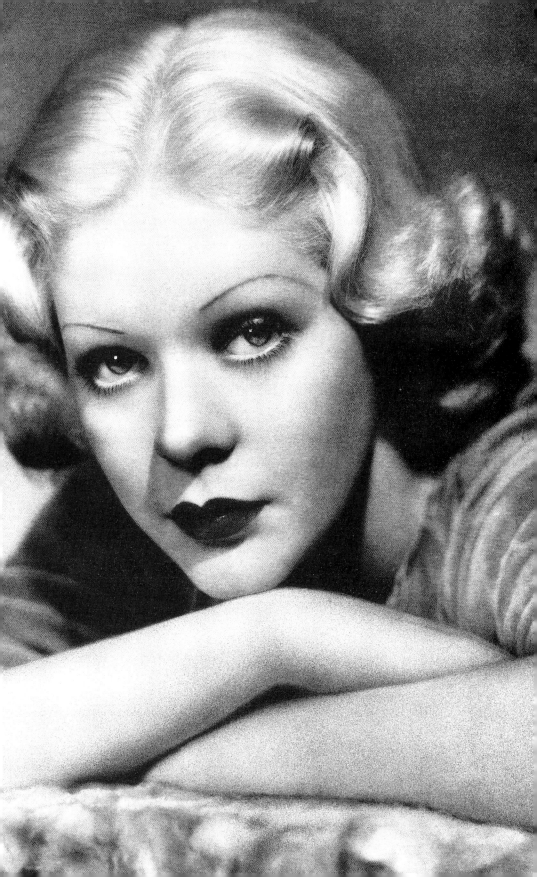

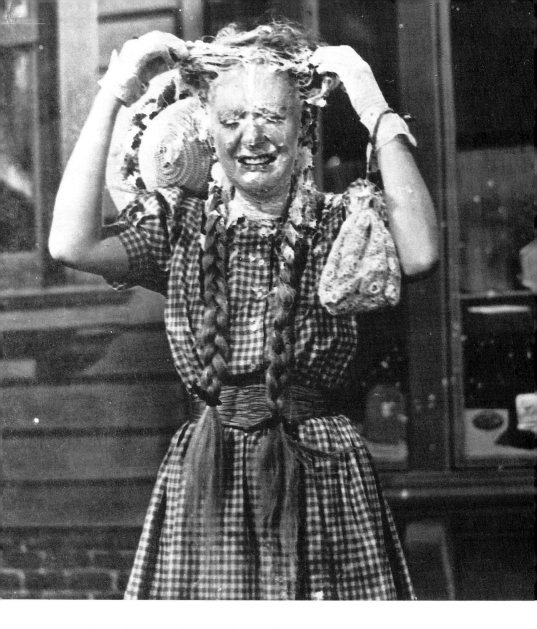

(ABOVE) *A scene from* Hollywood Cavalcade. *Alice's costars were Don Ameche and Buster Keaton.* (PHOTO COURTESY OF 20TH CENTURY–FOX)

(OPPOSITE) *Alice Faye starred in* In Old Chicago *with Don Ameche and Tyrone Power.*

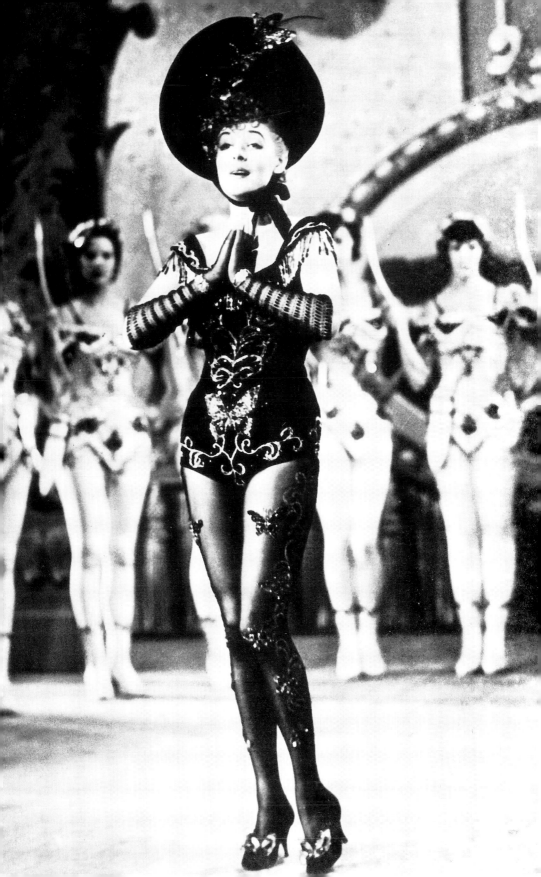

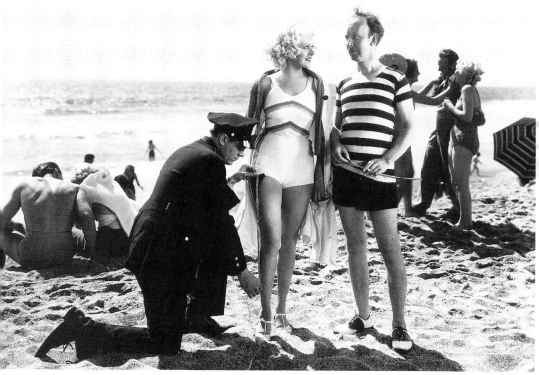

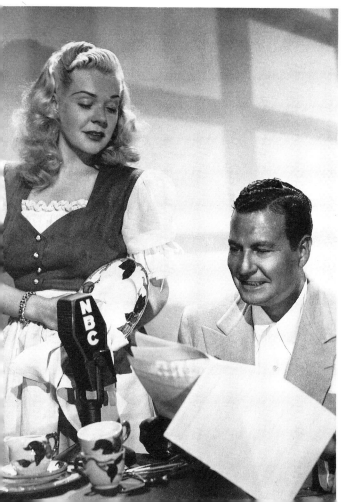

(ABOVE) *Alice Faye in* Now I'll Tell. (PHOTO COURTESY OF 20TH CENTURY–FOX)
(LEFT) *Alice Faye and Phil Harris on the set of their radio show.*

(OPPOSITE) *Alice Faye with President Dwight Eisenhower at a charity affair at Thunderbird Country Club.*

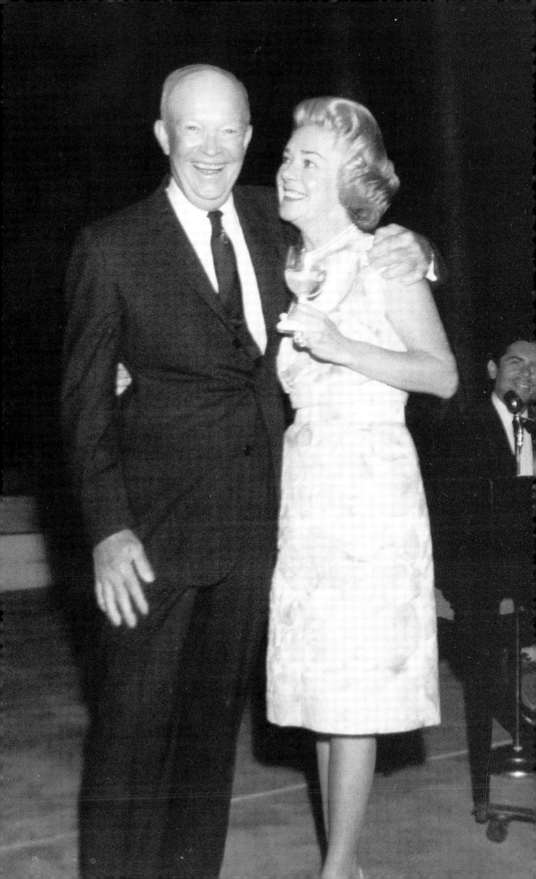

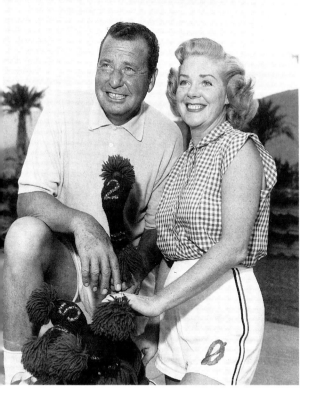

(LEFT) *Alice Faye and Phil Harris in front of their home at Thunderbird Country Club, 1952.* (PHOTO BY GAIL B. THOMPSON) (BELOW) *Alice Faye with Bing Crosby and Phil Harris.*

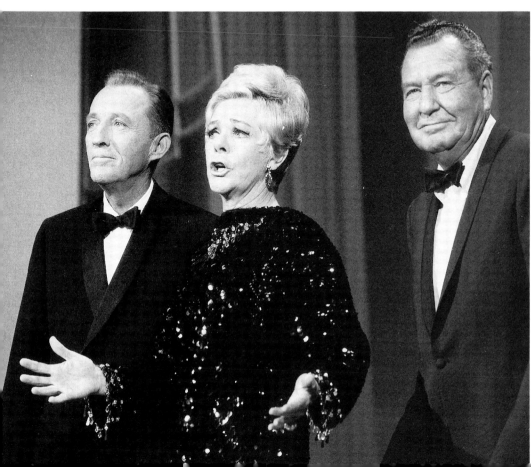

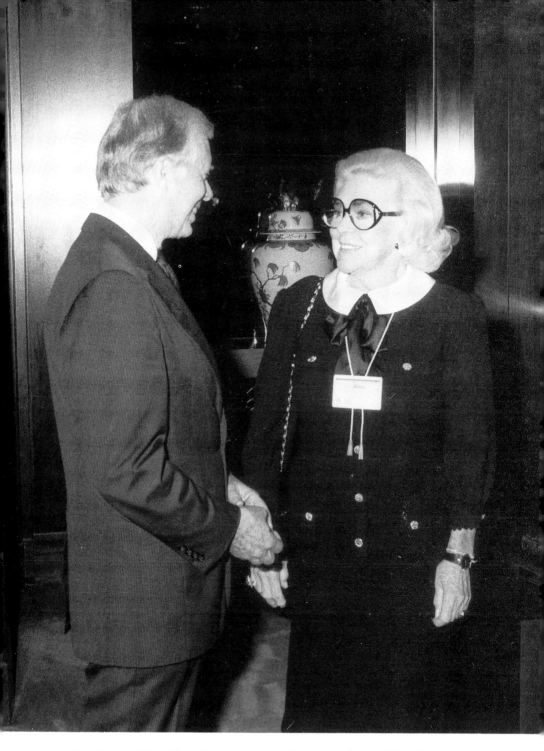

On the road for Pfizer Pharmaceuticals, here with President Jimmy Carter. (PHOTO COURTESY OF PFIZER PHARMACEUTICALS)

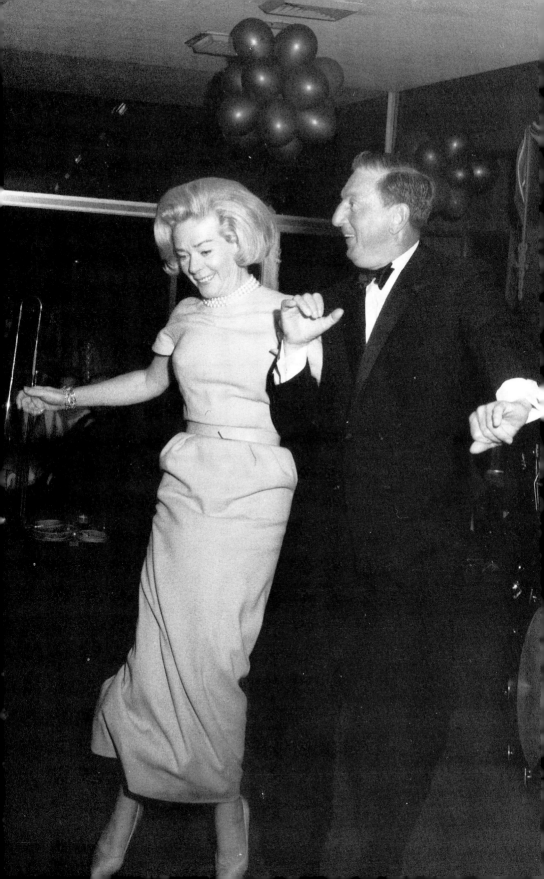

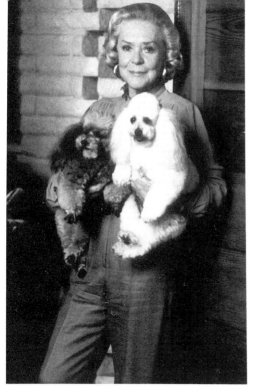

(OPPOSITE) *Dancing with Ray Bolger at a Thunderbird Country Club gala for a church charity, 1982.* (PHOTO BY MARK GLASSMAN)

(LEFT) *Alice Faye with Chula and Jessica at her home at the Thunderbird Country Club, 1982.* (BELOW) *Family portrait taken during the taping of "This Is Your Life, Alice Faye," 1984. Standing from left to right: daughter Phyllis, grandchildren Darren and Tammy, daughter Alice, grandson Gregory, Tony Gallo, and grandson Philip.*

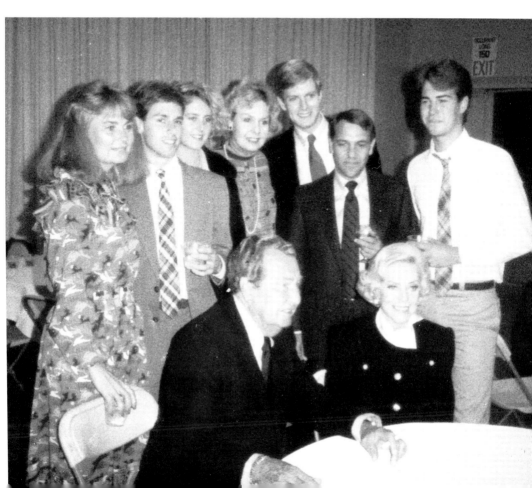

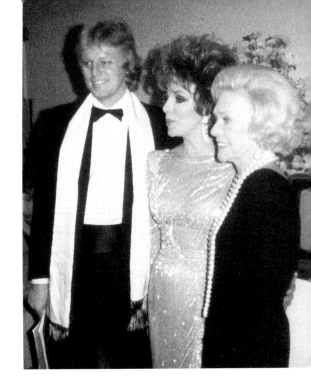

(CLOCKWISE FROM RIGHT) *Alice Faye in London for a benefit, here with Joan Collins and Peter Holm, 1985. Christmas party at Vintage Country Club in Palm Desert, 1986. Alice Faye with daughters Phyllis and Alice, 1987. Alice Faye and other celebrities being presented to Queen Elizabeth II at a charity event, 1985.*

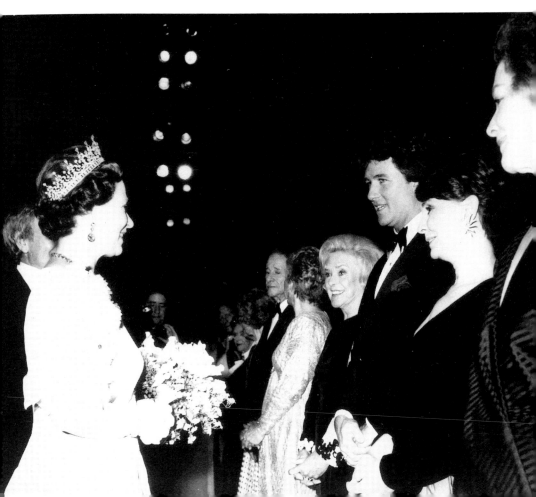

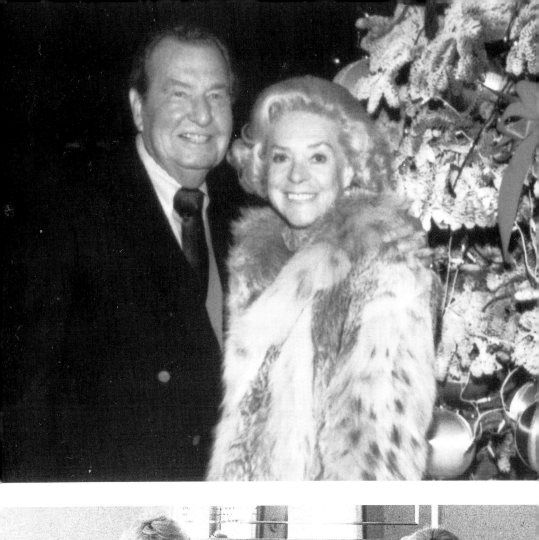

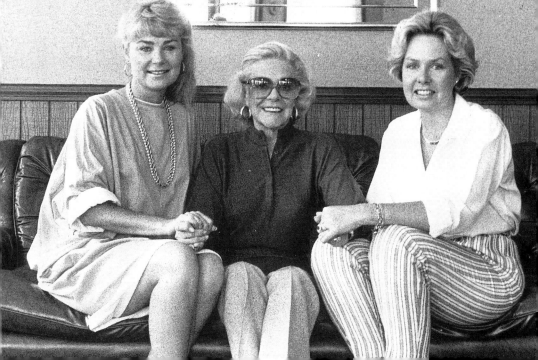

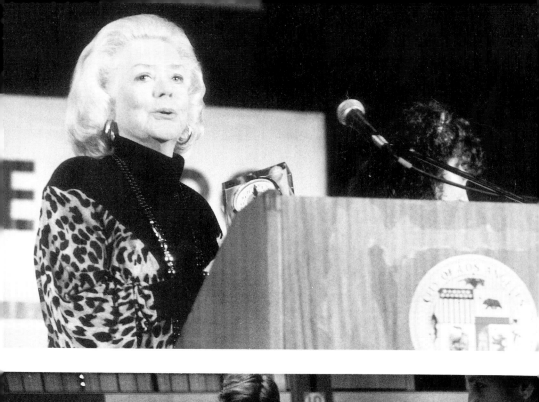

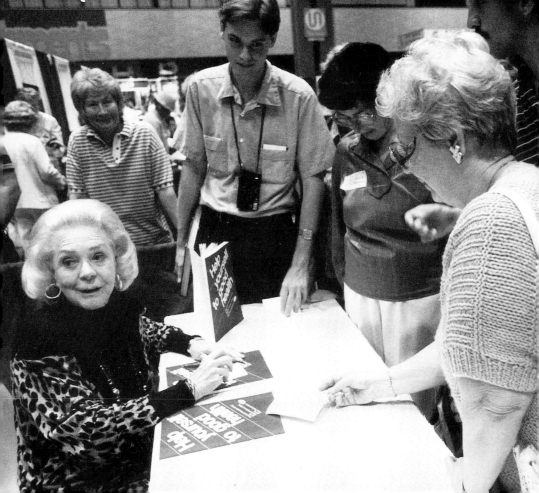

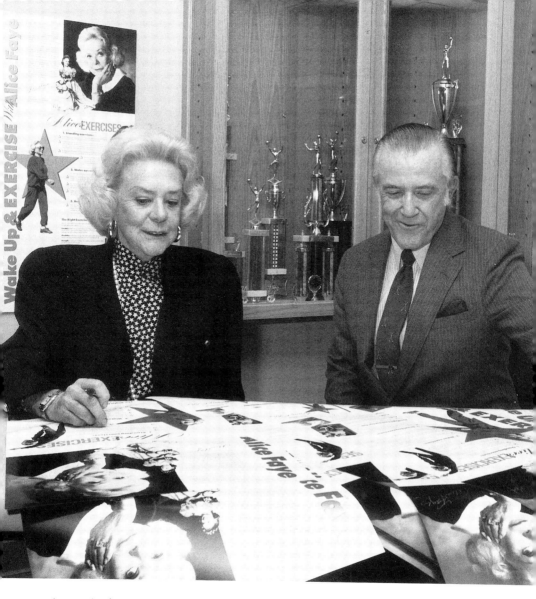

(ABOVE) *Alice Faye with Pfizer Pharmaceuticals' CEO, Edmund Pratt, Jr.*
(PHOTO COURTESY OF PFIZER PHARMACEUTICALS)

(OPPOSITE TOP) *Alice Faye speaking at the Los Angeles "Time of Your Life" Expo for Pfizer Pharmaceuticals, 1987.*
(OPPOSITE) *Alice Faye for Pfizer Pharmaceuticals, here with fans at the Los Angeles "Time of Your Life" Expo, 1987.*

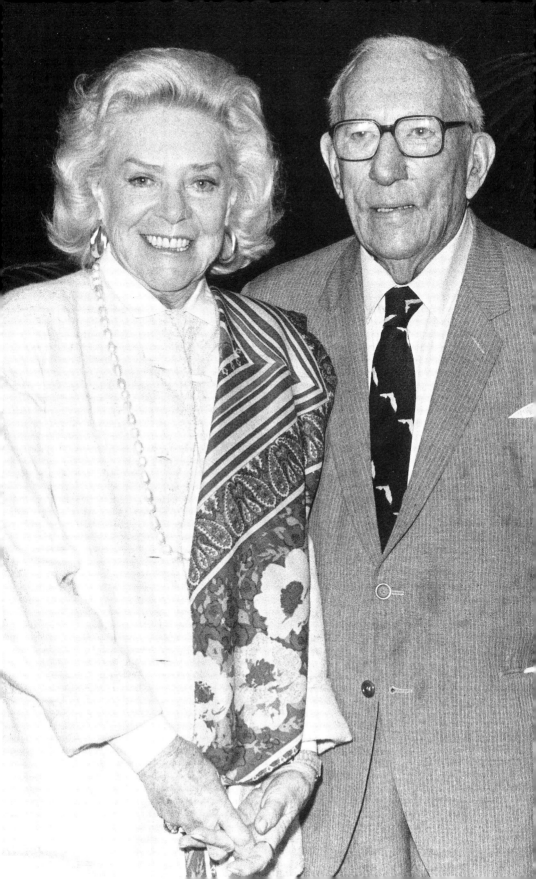

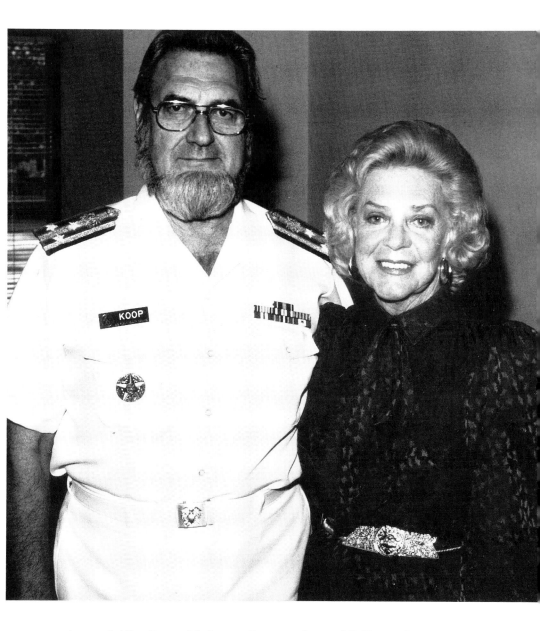

(ABOVE) *Alice Faye with former Surgeon General C. Everett Koop.* (PHOTO COURTESY OF PFIZER PHARMACEUTICALS)
(OPPOSITE) *Alice Faye with the late Honorable Claude Pepper.* (PHOTO COURTESY OF PFIZER PHARMACEUTICALS)

(OVERLEAF) *Phil Harris and Alice Faye doing their bit for the Cancer Society, which they do every year in Palm Desert.*

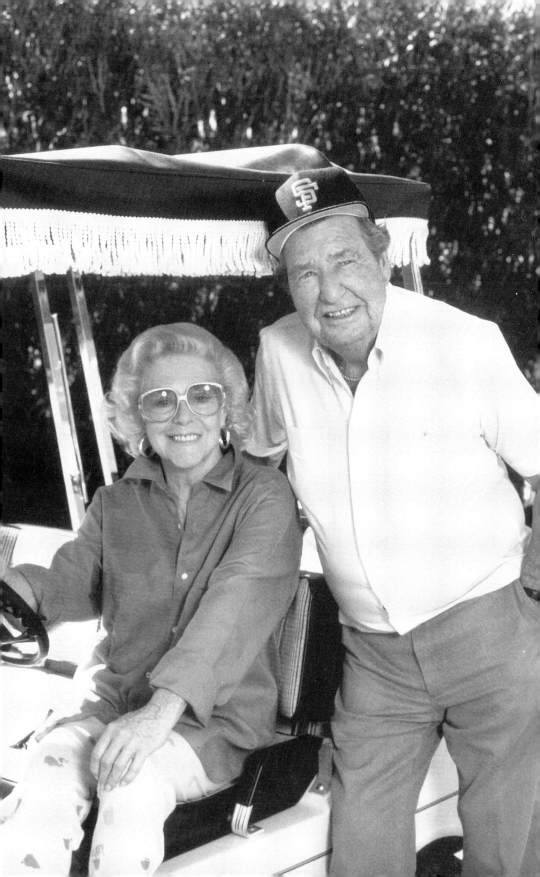

been consulting him for any length of time, he probably prescribed them originally—but it never hurts to remind him. "Doctor," you might say, as he hands you the new prescription, "this won't react badly with the pills I am taking for my insomnia, will it?" In ninety-nine cases out of a hundred, your doctor will say that, no, there is no problem, that he took your medication for insomnia into consideration when he prescribed the new high blood pressure medication. But there is always that hundredth case.

Never hesitate to ask your doctor a question. After all, it is a matter of life and death—and the life in question is yours, which is a pretty precious commodity.

Similarly, always tell your doctor if the drug he has prescribed is producing any unpleasant side effects—nausea, drowsiness, runny nose, whatever. He will start trying other drugs, or combinations of drugs, until you both settle on the one that is best for you. But, of course, your doctor won't know you are having a problem at all unless you tell him. So pick up the phone and say, "Gee, doctor, but that new medication seems to be giving me a buzzing in the ear," or whatever. And he will probably say something like, "It sometimes does produce that side effect, so let's try something else. I'll give your pharmacist a call with a new prescription. Let me know in a few days how that works for you."

You should be aware that pills to control your high blood pressure are not cheap. In fact, as drugs go, they are rather expensive. I estimate that my high blood pressure medication costs me a bit more than a dollar a day. In some family budgets that is a big bite. But you have to measure that expense against what it might cost if you were hospitalized with a stroke or a heart attack, and what it might cost for physical therapy after such a catastrophe, and what it might cost for nursing care or doctor care—or, God forbid, for a funeral. So, as someone once put it, maybe it's hard to afford to take the pills, but you can't afford not to take them.

One final precautionary note about blood pressure medicines. If you are taking them, be very careful when you take some other form of medication. You should be aware that some medicines you might innocently be taking—pills for allergies or colds or asthma, for example—can counteract the good the high blood pressure pills are doing. So don't take anything—either other prescription drugs or over-the-counter medications—without checking with your doctor.

ARTHRITIS: The next most common condition to afflict young elders is arthritis. I guess I am the typical young elder, because I also have a touch of arthritis too. It affects my hands and my lower back but, compared with many people's, my condition is mild, so I can't complain about it too vociferously. I may moan and groan a bit on those days when it is troubling me, but really it isn't too bad ordinarily. For some people, however, osteoarthritis—to give it its official name—can be a terrible thing. The pain can be so excruciating that the poor person who has it hates to move even an inch.

My brother, Charley, was very arthritic. I watched him suffer terrible pain. So, even though my own is mild, I know how rough it can be.

I just refuse to let my arthritis govern me. There are days when I would much prefer to just sit there quietly, without stirring, but that's the easy way out. And I refuse to confine myself to a chair, like an old lady. So I say to myself, "Alice, old girl, get yourself up and moving!" So I keep active, pain or not. And I get up and go out and walk or swim or both, and it's much better that way.

The weather, of course, affects my arthritis. Damp days are the worst. Sudden changes in weather can be brutal, too. That's when I really have to push myself to get up and keep moving.

Actually, when I said that osteoarthritis is the official name for arthritis, I was only partially correct. Science has identified several types of arthritis. Osteoarthritis is the name of the most common form, the one most people think of when they use the word "arthritis." But there are several other forms, and your doctor will tell you which one is yours.

Arthritis is a condition, as anyone who has it knows only too well, that affects the joints—ankles, knees, hips, fingers, wrists, anywhere in the body where two bones come together and are joined by cartilage. That cartilage is designed by nature to cover the bones at the joint, and make their movement smooth and painless. In arthritics, the cartilage has, for some reason, eroded away. Eventually it virtually disappears, so that you have two bones rubbing against each other without that protective coating. The result: *pain!*

Making the condition worse is the fact that, as the cartilage disappears, the bones develop spurs—little mounds or points—which aggravate the pain when the bones rub together.

Our grandparents and great-grandparents suffered from arthritis, but they simply considered it an inevitable part of the aging process. If they called it anything, they called it "rheumatism," which isn't really the same thing. But mostly they would hurt in the shoulder or in the hand and say, "Well, I must be getting old, after all." Today we know that it is osteoarthritis—and also that something can be done about it.

As with high blood pressure, or any other disease, for that matter, the sooner osteoarthritis is diagnosed and treatment begun, the better. If the disease is given a long time to develop in your body, it will be much more difficult to control. So don't hesitate to tell your doctor if you feel twinges of pain in any of your joints. Some people are reluctant to complain about their aches and pains, for fear they will be considered hypochondriacs. But it's much smarter, I think, to complain too often than to suffer needlessly. If it hurts, do something about it.

Osteoarthritis's first symptom, however, can be something other than pain. In fact, frequently the first sign of the disease is stiffness in the affected joint. So watch for that. Watch for waking up some morning and finding that it is tough to straighten out your arm because your elbow is stiff. If that happens a few days in a row, see your doctor.

Actually, from what doctors tell me, osteoarthritis is a baffling disease, in that it affects people so differently. Some may have severe pain from the start. Others may only have that condition of stiffness, with very little pain. And still others may have a stiffness in one joint and pain in another. So there are no hard and fast rules for osteoarthritis sufferers. Sometimes—as in my case—the pain is relatively mild. In others it grows progressively worse until it is crippling.

Although osteoarthritis is commonly believed to affect only people in their sixties and seventies, this is not true. The majority of sufferers are in that age bracket, but it is not uncommon for people in their thirties, forties, and fifties to find that they have osteoarthritis, too.

Who gets it? And why?

The answers to those questions are mostly theories. As with most diseases, science suspects now that heredity has a great great deal to do with the onset of osteoarthritis. Research has shown that some families are much more prone to developing osteoarthritis than others.

Another theory currently being advanced in scientific circles is that certain repeated physical activities can lead to arthritis. Although there are many exceptions to this theory, it does appear to be possible that football players, for example, who put a tremendous amount of strain on their knees, stand a good chance of winding up with arthritic knees in their later years.

So experts now say that, if you want to lessen your risk of arthritis as you grow older, don't put too much strain on any particular joint in your younger years. But this can be hard advice to follow if, for instance, your work includes some repeated use of a joint. Writers and secretaries, who use their fingers repeatedly in typing, can be considered at risk for arthritis in their hands. Punch press operators' elbows and shoulders are in use constantly, so they have a good chance of contracting arthritis in those joints as the years go by.

Determination of the causes of arthritis is still in the theoretical stage. What matters to most of us, however, isn't so much how we happened to get it, but what we can do about it. Leave the theory to the scientists, just help me with this pain!

In the first place, you can be sure to have it diagnosed properly and correctly. And that, of course, means a visit to your doctor's office and a thorough examination. The doctor will tell you which form of arthritis you have and what to do about it.

Arthritis, like most diseases, does not happen overnight. It's not like switching a light—now it's off, now it's on. It happens slowly, insidiously. A little stiffness here, a twinge of pain there. They come, they go. You think that maybe something is wrong, but you can't be sure. Days may go by without any problem, so that little stiffness may have been just a figment of your imagination. But then it comes back again, and this time it lingers a little longer and is a bit more severe, and this time it hurts, too.

The only way you can be sure is by telling your doctor what is happening, and letting him check you out thoroughly.

The doctor's first weapon in detecting whether or not you have arthritis is the X ray. This gives a picture of the affected joint and what's going on there. He may also draw out some of the fluid that the body produces to lubricate the joints. That fluid, examined under a microscope, will show signs of the onset of arthritis. As a basis of comparison the doctor may examine normal joints, too.

There are, as I have said, several types of arthritis. So one important conclusion your doctor will have to reach is what form—if any—you have. By far the most common is osteoarthritis, so let's assume that's what you have.

Like high blood pressure, osteoarthritis can be controlled but cannot be cured. As far as most of us are concerned, it is control that we desperately want—control over the pain and the stiffness so we can go on with our normal activities.

The way to control the pain is primarily through medication. Painkillers, beginning with good old reliable aspirin, are tried first. If they work, you can stick with them. But in many cases something stronger is indicated, so your doctor will suggest other over-the-counter painkillers, and then, if you still need more relief, progress to painkillers for which prescriptions are necessary. One way or another, your doctor will find something that will do the trick for you, and lessen the pain.

If the pain is particularly intense, your doctor may give you a shot of cortisone. When injected directly into the affected joint, cortisone works wonders. It may initially seem to heighten the pain, but that is temporary. After a day or so the pain magically goes away. But the problem with cortisone—which is a steroid—is that it can cause an adverse reaction. Furthermore, the relief it provides is only temporary; more cortisone shots produce greater side effects; and each shot results in relief that lasts for a shorter and shorter period. So cortisone is a last resort.

Besides the painkiller your doctor may prescribe one of several drugs designed to reduce inflammation. Inflammation is a by-product of arthritis caused by the constant rubbing of joints, unprotected by sufficient cartilage. Antiinflammatory drugs will reduce that condition, lessening at least some of the pain.

Medication is only part of the arthritis control program your doctor will probably suggest for you. He most likely will also want you to begin a series of exercises designed to strengthen the affected joint and the muscles around it. At the same time, the doctor will probably advise you to give that poor joint of yours some rest. It may sound contradictory—to suggest both exercise and rest for the same joint—but there is a point to doing both.

You must exercise the joint, because if you don't you run the very serious risk of having it freeze up on you, so you lose its use permanently. Remember the old motto Use It or Lose It. Your doctor will want to make sure you don't lose it, so he will insist you use it. By "exercise," the doctor doesn't mean anything overly strenuous; probably just to move the affected joint as much as you can. Suppose it is a shoulder that is troubling you. Your doctor will advise you to move your arm as far as it will go in every direction, thus putting your shoulder through its entire range of motion. If it is a hip, the doctor will want you to move your leg back and forth, and from side to side, again making the joint move in every direction it's meant to.

If it seems to be impossible for you to do anything of this sort yourself, your doctor may suggest that you see a physical therapist for a round of what are called "passive exercises." In these, someone else moves your limb for you, thus giving that joint some exercise. The hope is that eventually you will be able to do the motions for yourself again.

Naturally, if it is at all possible, you should do your own exercising. In fact, although nobody can say for sure at this point, there is a large body of respected medical opinion that believes that proper exercising can prevent arthritis. Certainly if you put each of your joints through its entire range of motion every day—doing some of the exercises I talk about in Chapter 7—you stand a good chance of escaping the worst forms of arthritis.

But rest is equally important. The idea is to strike a balance between exercise and rest. Too much exercise is just as bad as too little. Some experts advise a period of rest after each exercise session that is as long as the period of exercise. If you exercise a half hour, they say, you should follow that up with a half-hour rest period. By rest they do not mean you have to lie down and go to sleep. Simply sitting comfortably and reading or contemplating your navel qualifies as rest. The point is to let the joint have some time off.

Another seemingly contradictory method of treatment for arthritic pain is the use of both hot and cold applications. It all depends on what feels good to you. Neither heat nor cold will cure arthritis, but both have been known to offer some temporary relief from its pain. (If you do use heat, please be careful—it is easy to overdo it, and suffer burns as a result.) So try both, and if it feels good to have a heating pad on your poor, aching elbow, by all means use it. Or if an ice pack seems to do a better job of deadening the pain, then keep that ice handy.

A lot of people find that dunking their whole pain-ridden body in a hot bathtub is pure bliss. And others find an ice-cold shower makes them forget the pain. So do whatever feels best to you.

When my arthritis acts up, mostly in my fingers and hands, I find that the best thing is to keep busy. Being active takes my mind off my pain. If you succumb to it, and sit around and brood about it, the pain can get worse and worse. I may take a Tylenol if it is particularly severe, but I try not to, because I don't like to take too much medication. (I checked with my doctor, and he said a Tylenol once in a while was OK.)

I believe that both my poodles have arthritis, too. They are getting on—one is eight and one is twelve—and sometimes they lie around and seem to have a lot of trouble standing up. So the three of us are quite a trio. I try to help them stand up and move around, and I think doing that helps me, too.

I also find I get some relief from the pain in my fingers

and my hands by squeezing a hard rubber ball. I keep it beside my table, with my book, and when I read I pick it up and squeeze away. I also carry it with me when I travel, and I've seen my seatmates on planes do a double take when I reach into my purse, pull out my little rubber ball, and start squeezing it. It seems to help me a lot, so I'll keep on squeezing no matter how odd it looks to other people.

I love to do needlepoint, too. And it is a curious thing, but sometimes that activity helps soothe my painful fingers. At other times, however, it seems to aggravate the pain. I can never be sure, when I pick up my current project, if it is going to make my fingers hurt more or feel better.

Someone once suggested to me that I should try acupuncture for my arthritis. But if there is one thing I'm a coward about, it's getting stuck with needles. So I passed on acupuncture and cannot offer any personal knowledge about whether it is of value, although some people swear by it.

There are other forms of treatment for arthritis. Some are so new—such as the use of ultrasound—that the medical jury is still out on their efficacy. Others are so old—surgery, for example—that current thought considers them of little relevance in today's medical arsenal. Today, most doctors look on surgery as a last resort in the treatment of arthritis. Only if a joint is so crippled by the disease that it is actually ossified will they consider an operation to replace it. Such operations are possible but so drastic that doctors today prefer any reasonable alternative.

Let's move on to another disease that frequently affects us young elders. This is diabetes. I am fortunate in that I do not have any sign of it—knock on wood.

DIABETES: Like the other diseases we have discussed in this chapter, diabetes is controllable but not curable. And, again like high blood pressure and arthritis, the sooner it is detected the better the chances that it can be effectively controlled.

Your doctor, during your regular physical checkup, will almost certainly ask for blood and urine tests. These detect the first signs of incipient diabetes.

"Well," your doctor will say, "it looks like we have a small problem." (There's that "we" again!) The doctor will say your blood sugar count is elevated above normal limits. He or she will explain about diabetes, a dangerous disease if left unchecked. In a body that is operating normally, a gland called the pancreas produces insulin, a hormone that helps the body take glucose from the bloodstream and turn it into useful material—cells that go to make up muscles and brain matter, for example. In diabetics, the pancreas doesn't produce enough insulin to do the job, or (as some researchers now believe) the insulin it does produce is in some way inferior. In either case the upshot is that the body, without enough top-grade insulin, is no longer making the cells it needs to function smoothly. A sure sign that this is occurring is when the blood sugar level rises drastically, indicating that the glucose is staying in the bloodstream rather than being transferred into useful cells.

Diabetes is a progressive disease and eventually may result in death. The good news is that it can be controlled. Shots supply the insulin the pancreas is not making. But today even those shots may not be necessary—provided the disease is spotted early enough. Now there are oral drugs that control the level of blood sugar. If the disease progresses, of course, insulin may become necessary, but many people can avoid this by taking these other drugs.

At the time your doctor prescribes these drugs, he or she will also place you on a strict diet. Obviously, if your body can't handle sugar it is only logical that you must keep your sugar intake down to a minimum. No point in adding to the body's difficulties. You will be told to avoid all foods that contain sugar, and that doesn't merely mean lemon meringue pie and tollhouse cookies. Many other foods are chock-full of sugar, as you will find out when your doctor gives you the list of foods to avoid.

Is there any way to prevent diabetes from striking you? Most scientists are convinced that this is a hereditary disease. So if there is a history of diabetes in your family tree, it is a good idea to have your blood and urine checked more often than other people do.

It also makes sense, if you wish to avoid diabetes in your later years, to go easy on the amount of sugar you consume. Don't put four or five heaping spoonfuls of sugar into your coffee or on your morning cereal. Even a pancreas that is operating normally has a tough time handling all that sugar.

Other than take these precautions, about the only thing you can do is cross your fingers. But, of course, make it a point to see your doctor regularly so if diabetes attacks you can detect it early.

Recent studies seem to indicate that exercise may be helpful in treating diabetes. Nobody knows why, but diabetics test out with lower blood sugar levels after an exercise session than they do immediately before.

Of course, it has long been known that obese people have a tougher time fighting diabetes than thin people. For some reason the insulin works more slowly—and sometimes, fatally, not at all—in people who are grossly overweight. So that is another reason to stay as slim as possible.

CANCER: Finally, of course, there is cancer. This terrible disease comes in so many types and attacks so many parts of the body that I can't possibly discuss them all. But cancer differs in one dramatic way from the other conditions I have just discussed. Cancer, if detected soon enough, can be cured.

For centuries, cancer was the most dreaded of all diseases, because it was an automatic death sentence. But we are living in the best of all times—so far—and today many forms of cancer can be defeated outright. Early detection, however, is the key to that defeat.

Cancer means that certain cells begin—for reasons science still does not understand—to go wild. They grow at an uncontrollable rate. If their growth is left unchecked, these cancerous cells eventually spread throughout the body (a process called metastasis), and death is the inevitable result. But nowadays, in many types of cancer, that growth can be checked and often completely stopped.

One of the most common forms of cancer—cancer of the rectum—is a good example of the progress medicine has made in cancer treatment. Today, if cancer of the rectum is detected soon enough, it can be cured in 75 percent of all cases. But it all hinges on those words—"If it is detected soon enough."

The key, of course, is regular trips to the doctor and being something of a doctor's assistant yourself. You have to tell the doctor if there is anything that seems suspicious to you. Don't hesitate to mention any unusual goings-on with your body. And be aware of the cancer danger signs.

If you have a cough that persists, tell your doctor. A prolonged cough could be an indication of lung cancer. Similarly, if you cough up blood. Or if you are constantly short of breath.

In women, of course, even a tiny lump in the breast may be a sign of cancer. Doctors or clinics will show you how to examine your breasts for cancer symptoms. Breast cancer can strike women of any age—there have even been cases of teenage girls who contracted it. But it generally strikes women over thirty. Actually, the heaviest incidence is in the fifty-nine-to-seventy-nine age bracket. According to a chart I recently saw compiled by SEER Data, almost four women out of one thousand in that age category were diagnosed as having breast cancer. So it behooves women of all ages to keep a careful eye on any changes in their breasts.

If your bowel habits change markedly, that could be an indication of cancer of the colon or rectum. Similarly, blood in your stool is something you should mention to your doctor.

For men over a certain age, cancer of the prostate is a common affliction. Watch for changes in urinating habits—if urination causes pain, or if you find you have to urinate more frequently than usual, especially at night.

If you have any sores on your body that fail to heal after a reasonable length of time, they could be a symptom of melanoma, or other forms of cancer. Watch, too, for any changes in the color or size of any moles you may have.

Women should also be wary of bleeding after menopause or any peculiar vaginal discharges, both of which can be signs of cancer of the uterus, ovaries, or cervix.

Tell your doctor if you notice any of these symptoms, or anything else that seems strange to you.

Even if you don't have such symptoms, you could be getting cancer, and your doctor will probably perform certain procedures and tests to help detect any incipient cancer developing. Rectal exams, annoying and uncomfortable as they are, are important in this regard. For women, pelvic exams and Pap tests are vital.

If a cancer is pinpointed early in its development, it can be cured in more and more cases. The method may vary. It could be surgery to remove, say, a skin cancer. Or it could be treatment via drugs, called chemotherapy. Or radiation therapy.

So never hesitate to mention to your doctor that something is troubling you. Maybe it's only a tiny pimple that has popped up inside your mouth and doesn't seem to go away. Or a little lump on your back. Maybe it's nothing. Maybe it's something. If it's something, chances are good that it can be taken care of, so it will never amount to SOMETHING. Maybe it can be handled by minor surgery, maybe by drugs, maybe by any number of the ways of treating cancers that science is discovering every day.

But the thing to remember here is that if you want to Grow Older but Stay Young you first have to grow older. And the only way to do that is to stick around. And to do that you must detect and treat and therefore control those diseases that commonly afflict us as we get older. Making our bodies as healthy as possible is the essential first step to staying young.

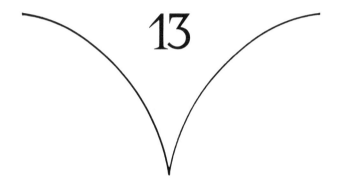

13

People have been concerned about being beautiful (or handsome, depending on their sex) since ancient times. The Egyptians knew and used cosmetics, and the Greeks and Romans were vain about their looks. Plutarch wrote one of my all-time favorite quotations, "When the candles are out, all women are fair," so it's clear that the subject of beauty even concerned ancient philosophers.

Down through the centuries, in virtually every civilization on every continent, being beautiful (or handsome) has been considered a worthy goal in life. It doesn't matter if it is the African tribe who stick plates in their lips or the Eskimos who tattoo their noses, we all do what we have to to look our best.

Perhaps our civilization places too high a value on beauty. But that is another question, certainly not one I am going to get into in this book. We are stuck here, in this particular civilization, and we have to play by its rules and try to get along as best we can.

So you want to look your best. It was a lot easier to do that when you had youth on your side. At eighteen and twenty you could stay up all night, hop out of bed the next morning, comb your hair, put on a bit of lipstick and makeup, and look pretty good.

I never spent much time on makeup and such, unless, of course, I was going to step in front of the camera. And then there was a battery of makeup men and hairstylists to assist me, so I really never paid much attention to doing my face. I used to boast that, as far as makeup was concerned, I was pretty much a soap-and-water gal. I was blessed with a good complexion and good coloring—fair skin, blue eyes, and blond hair were always considered "good"—so I didn't have to do much more than keep it all clean and neat.

When I first signed with 20th Century–Fox, as I said earlier, they thought I could be another Jean Harlow. She was at the peak of her brief career then—she died in 1937, a few years after I began in the movies—and success always breeds imitations. Darryl Zanuck felt that there was room for another platinum-blond bombshell, and he had the idea that he could transform me into one.

So for a time I was a platinum blonde. The studio makeup department changed my makeup to match my hair coloring and plucked my eyebrows into skinny little lines, and during those few years I did wear a lot of powder, rouge, mascara, and the whole bit. I always felt, at night, as though I had to peel my face off before I got down to the real me.

Happily, that only lasted a few years and a few pictures. The studio brass eventually decided that I could go back to my natural hair coloring—blond, but not the dazzling platinum sort of blond—and makeup to match. Their decision made me much more comfortable. The last picture in which

I was burdened with "the Harlow look" was *Poor Little Rich Girl* in 1936. After that I was able to unpluck my eyebrows and tell the studio hairdressing department to deep-six the bottle of peroxide.

My next picture was *Stowaway*, and, in that, my hair is roughly my natural color and my eyebrows are normal, and that's the way I looked pretty much from then on.

Through the years I have occasionally touched up my hair with coloring. In one way, we blondes have the edge on brunettes: as our hair becomes gray, the difference between what once was and what now is just isn't so startling. When a brunette shows gray, everybody notices immediately and comments. But a blonde can go gray gradually and the change is barely noticeable. In fact, I haven't done a thing to the coloring of my hair in five years. I just let it age in a natural way.

So as I grew older I grew grayer, but that alone did not drastically alter my appearance. And I did not wrinkle as badly as some men and women do. I have my share of wrinkles, but they are not deep crevices. That's mostly a matter of luck.

I think I was also blessed with the sense to understand a few basic truths about the fine art of makeup.

For one thing, makeup is not a substitute for beauty. Nor is it a way to cover or mask the aging process. If you are beginning to show the signs of the advancing years, you can't slap on an extra-heavy coating of makeup and think you have, willy-nilly, covered up those signs. It doesn't work that way. As a matter of fact, the older we get, the less war paint we ladies should use. Nothing looks more pitiful than an older woman with a thick coating of rouge, layers and layers of eye shadow, and thick lines of mascara and lipstick spread on with a spatula.

I see a poor lady like that and I could weep for her. If she only knew that, without all that glop on her face, she would look so much younger and more attractive. But she puts it on in a vain attempt to recapture her lost youth, which is beyond recapture no matter how much makeup she uses.

Actually, using too much makeup only calls attention to wrinkles and other signs of aging. So if you want to look younger than you are, the first lesson is to go easy on all forms of makeup. Use it, but use it judiciously.

I tell women that there is a similarity between getting makeup advice and seeing a doctor. When you want to make sure you *feel* your best, you should see a doctor regularly and follow his or her directions to the letter. When you want to make sure you *look* your best, you should see a makeup specialist. You don't need to see him, or her, regularly—once every five or six years will probably suffice—but you should follow the advice the makeup specialist gives you to the letter, too.

Few women are their own best makeup experts. It is very tough to be objective about your appearance. That is why a makeup expert is essential. The expert is totally objective. He or she probably has never seen you before and probably will never see you again. You are just a passing face, so the specialist can tell you what is best for you without any prejudice or preconceived notions.

You will find makeup experts at the better beauty salons and at the cosmetics counters in the leading department stores. I have found that the cosmetics sections of the better department stores almost always have very competent experts who will show you what sort of makeup is best for your face, at your age. These services are usually inexpensive, and sometimes they are free, assuming you make a purchase from the department. The experts you talk with will undoubtedly recommend products that they have for sale, which, of course, is only sound commercial practice. But there is no law that says you have to buy from them; you can take their recommendations and go next door where the prices are cheaper and buy the same things, or reasonably accurate equivalents.

The point is that every few years, I believe, we all need some professional makeup advice. After I left the studio, I continued to use basically the same sort of makeup. After all, the Hollywood set makeup experts are the finest in the world, so I would have been foolish to try something different. I was fortunate to have the fabulous Westmores taking care of my makeup. Those Westmore brothers were the best in the business, and they worked at most of the major studios. Many Hollywood stars became so attached to, and dependent on, their makeup people that they would insist on them going along when they traveled or when they were loaned out to other studios. That applied to men as well as women—both Bob Hope and Bing Crosby had their personal makeup men and wouldn't leave home without them. I didn't, because I knew that the Westmores—one or more of them, and to me they were practically interchangeable—would be around to give me the finest possible makeup and makeup advice.

Of course, being the young leading lady throughout my entire career, I never wore extreme makeup. And even though my character might have lived a long life—which happened in films such as *Alexander's Ragtime Band* and *Lillian Russell*—I was not allowed to show my age. The plot line of *Alexander's Ragtime Band* spanned several decades, but neither Tyrone Power nor I showed any signs of those advancing years. That was the way it was in Hollywood in those days—the stars had to look glamorous no matter how old they were supposed to be.

But even within Hollywood's dictates, the Westmores worked makeup miracles. And I still basically follow the advice they gave me then. I use much less makeup nowadays, of course, because you need more when you are on camera, but the same principles apply.

Perhaps five or six years after I left the studio, I felt I had changed enough that it was time to revise my makeup system. I went to an expert and had my makeup redesigned. I have done that every five or six years or so since then. It seems to me that this is roughly the right time frame for everyone. Our faces don't change so swiftly that we need makeup help any more often. But the change is inexorable, and we must recognize that fact.

Some of us change more than others. Some of us change in little ways, barely discernible. But everyone changes. Some may notice that their eyelashes have begun to fade. That is often one of the first symptoms of age, particularly in women with brunette or dark brown lashes. That's when it's time to get out the old mascara—a little touch and the eyes look better, brighter.

Eyebrows, too, tend to change their shape. The eyebrows are an oft-neglected part of our facial anatomy, yet they are so important to appearance. Touch them up if they have paled. If you dye your hair, don't leave your eyebrows out in the cold. In most of us the color of our hair matches the color of our eyebrows. So if you change one, change the other. If your eyebrows have gotten too thin with the passage of time, thicken then with the judicious application of eyebrow pencil. If they have thickened, pluck them—not too much, just enough so they are under control.

You may find yourself wearing eyeglasses now. If you do—this is a tip from the Westmores—wear a bit heavier eye makeup than you formerly did. Eyeglasses have a tendency to diminish the effect of eye makeup, so you have to counteract that tendency.

On most of us, our cheeks tend to pale over the years. A bit of blush—not too heavy, of course—restores the color we all need to look our best. This may sound like I am contradicting myself—earlier I said use less makeup as you age—but here I am talking mostly to those healthy, sun-kissed women who seldom used any makeup at all. These ladies may need a bit of help as they get older and their complexions grow paler.

Lips, too, may need more assistance. Too many women think all they have to do to their lips is daub a coat of lipstick over them. To make your lips look their best, first outline them with a lipstick pencil, then use lipstick. You'll find that outlining gives your lips a definition that is very attractive.

Most of us can use some help with our hair as we get on in years. An annual hairstyling may be in order. Or perhaps you don't need help that frequently. In fact, many women find a hairstyle they like, one they believe is flattering as well as comfortable, and they may stick with it the rest of their lives. Others like a change from time to time, or feel that a change is needed to make them look younger.

Hairstylists, like makeup experts, are objective, and, assuming you find one whose taste you like, you can rely on his or her good judgment and skill.

I have pretty much worn my hair the same way since I was a teenager. Even when it was dyed a flashy platinum shade, the style was virtually the same as it is today. It's either combed to the side or pulled back, but the length is the same either way. Once, for the fun of it, I had my hair cut quite short, but I never liked that; it simply did not feel comfortable on my head, and I let it grow back as quickly as nature would permit.

I actually prefer it when my hair is pulled back. I try not to let it get too long. Still, I like it long enough so I can pull it back easily. That, to me, is the most comfortable, and that's how my hair is when I'm at home and when I'm swimming and when I go marketing and for all my ordinary activities. But I wear it a bit shorter when I go traveling or go to any sort of public function. I think it looks a bit smarter at that length.

You should wear your hair the way you think it looks best, but if you have any doubts, don't ask the lady next door, ask a professional.

Whatever you do, don't try to keep up with the kids in the way you style your hair. Outlandish styles—such as the punk styles of today—are fine for teenagers. They're welcome to them. But nothing looks worse than a middle-aged lady (or beyond) who thinks she can keep up with her daughter or granddaughter and wears her hair in a teenage style. That poor lady winds up looking totally ridiculous. There is an age gap, after all, and you can't bridge it by aping teenage styles.

I believe strongly that for most women wild hairstyles detract from their natural beauty. Hair is, in a sense, the frame around a painting. If the painting is beautiful, having a terribly ornate frame only makes the eye look at the frame rather than the painting. The same applies to hairstyle; if you wear your hair in a fancy, fussy, frilly style, anyone you meet will look at your hair instead of your face.

If you have a beautiful face, then the whoop-de-doo hairstyle just draws attention away from your face. And if your face is anywhere from average through plain to not so hot, having a wild and woolly coiffure will only make you look ridiculous. So ornate hairdos help nobody. Stay away from them. Don't do a beehive or cornrows or anything that eye-catching unless you think your face is so ugly you want people to look at your hair, not your face. If you're that bad off, nothing really helps. Except maybe a paper bag.

What about dyeing your hair? Sure, why not? Here's a tip that I learned in my days in the studio—if you use hair coloring, try two different shades. They should be close to each other but not identical. The reason is that most hair naturally consists of two or more shades. So using the two hair colors gives your hair a much more natural look.

But don't run to the cosmetics counter and buy some hair coloring as soon as you spot that first gray hair on your head.

Think about letting it turn gray naturally. Actually, gray can be a very becoming color. Not for all women, of course, but for many. But if you think it is not a flattering shade for you, by all means color your hair. One suggestion I picked up at the studio: Never use a color that is darker than your original hair color. Go a shade or two lighter than the original. You'll see that it works.

The foundation on which all beauty and good looks are built is the skin. Men and women alike must have clean, healthy skin if they want to look their best, and this is true no matter what age you are or what other attributes you may or may not have. Somebody once estimated that your skin actually weighs more than your brain or, for that matter, any other organ in your body. There is a lot of skin out there, and many people take it for granted and/or abuse it dreadfully.

To begin with, as I just said, skin must be kept clean. This is especially important on your face, because that is the section of your skin that people see. When you meet people, it is your face they see first, so keep your best skin forward. Scrub your face well, morning and night. Use high-quality soap; don't cut corners by buying cheap stuff, because the difference in cost between good soap and cheap soap is minimal, but the difference between a good complexion and one that is spotty could be devastating to your life.

As we get older, our skin changes. There is really no way to prevent these changes; they are the wondrous workings of nature. We can, however, minimize the damage they wreak on our skin.

What are these changes? The primary one is that as we age our skin has a tendency to dry out. There are glands that produce the oils in our skin. When we are young, these glands go all out; thus, youthful skin is moist and well lubricated. But over the years these glands produce less and less oil. As a result our skin becomes dryer and dryer. (For a few people, whose skin was overly oily when they were young, this slowdown of oil production is a blessing, but for most people it is the opposite.)

At the same time that the skin receives less and less oil, another change is taking place. Our skin cells have a tendency, as we age, to alter their composition somewhat. I am not a physiologist (among many other things that I am not), so I don't pretend to understand everything that goes on. All I know is that my doctor friends tell me our skin cells later in life lose their ability to absorb and hold moisture.

It's kind of a double whammy. Our skin doesn't get as much oil from the glands as it once did, and our skin cells can't handle the oil they do get. Anyhow, the result is bad news. Our skin dries out, and dryness is why so many older people have skin that looks like the hide of a particularly nasty rhinoceros. We must counteract that tendency to dry skin. This is an essential first step if we are to Grow Older but Stay Young. It is impossible to stay young with skin that is fast turning into rhinoceros hide.

You will find many suggested ways of recapturing the skin's moisture. Some people advocate a large batch of vitamins. Some push all kinds of creams and lotions. Some say that exercise is beneficial, since it makes the body increase its intake of oxygen. They theorize that oxygen, because it is a component of water, is helpful in creating moisture in the body.

My own theory is that the skin is like your garden. If there is a dry spell, and your petunias and marigolds look thirsty, you water them. The same, I believe, holds true for your skin. If it is dry, water it. Wash it a couple of times a day, splash water on it in between washings, go swimming and submerge your face, shower and turn your face up to the nozzle so it gets a good soaking. And drink those six glasses of water a day, so you lubricate from the inside out, too. If it makes your face feel good to use some of those moisturizing creams or lotions, by all means use them. They can't hurt.

But, basically, just keep everything as moist as possible.

My skin is, I think, as moist as it can be, and I attribute much of that to the frequent swims I take. Of course, chlorine in swimming pools has the opposite effect—it tends to dry out the skin. (You just can't win!) So, while the swimming moistens, the chlorine dries. Moisturizers and, I believe, my massages help to balance the equations.

The dryness of skin is one factor in another calamity of aging—the coming of the wrinkle. People wrinkle at different speeds. Some begin to show wrinkles in their forties, others not until their sixties. Some wrinkle fast and deep, others slow and shallow. Some lucky ones, in their eighties, have relatively smooth skin, while others look like their faces have been crumpled like sheets of paper. What causes these differences? Nobody knows for sure; it is probably not any one thing but a combination of many factors.

Heredity, and with it ethnic origin, probably plays a large role in the wrinkling mechanism. Some nationalities appear to be relatively wrinkle proof whereas others are wrinkle prone. And the tendency to wrinkle also seems to run in some families more than others.

How much your face is exposed to wind, rain, sun, and all those natural forces is also important. We all have a picture in our mind's eye of the sailor or lumberjack, with his weather-beaten face—well, "weather-beaten" is just a euphemism for wrinkled. That sailor and that lumberjack, spending all their time outdoors, have their skin battered by the elements. That battering causes wrinkles. And even if you are neither a sailor nor a lumberjack but spend a lot of time outside, you will most likely wind up with more wrinkles than if you spend your time indoors in an office or a shop or your home. The great outdoors is the great enemy of a smooth skin.

Another way we can abuse our skin, and produce premature wrinkling, is intermittent dieting. Skin is something like a road, which expands in the summer heat, contracts in the winter cold, and, as a result, cracks and produces potholes. If we diet—thus contracting our skin—and then eat a lot and grow heavy again—thus expanding our skin—what is our skin to do but wrinkle in protest?

Some theorize that any abuse of the body—smoking too heavily, drinking too much, taking drugs—is also bound to have an adverse effect on the skin and make for early wrinkling. One of those abuses of the body you must be aware of is the lack of sufficient sleep. You know how you look when you haven't had enough sleep—like the wrath of God, as my grandmother used to say.

Back at the studio I worked in a film called *Music Is Magic,* in 1935, with Bebe Daniels. She was an old-timer in Hollywood—she had worked in silents, and she had been Harold Lloyd's leading lady—so she was no chicken then. But her skin was still a thing of beauty. One day I went to see her in her dressing room for something, and she was taking a nap.

"Don't you feel well, Bebe?" I asked her.

"Oh, I'm fine," she said. "Just taking my complexion nap."

She explained that she took naps whenever she could, because she felt doing so was beneficial to her skin. She was right. Doctors today say that lack of sleep harms the circulation, and it is good circulation that keeps the skin cells moist and fresh. So lack of sleep can contribute to circles under your eyes and a generally poor complexion.

When I was a child and made a face, my mother used to say, "If you keep making that face, your face is going to freeze like that." Well, our faces may not freeze in any set position, but if we do make the same facial expressions repeatedly, the skin will react by forming wrinkles along the lines of those expressions. If we frown, we will have frown lines. If we smile, laugh lines. And so on. So you should try to avoid forcing your face into any one expression too often.

If you find that some constant repetition of a facial expression is causing a line to appear, you can do something to cancel it out. If it is detected soon enough, you can make a point of adopting a facial expression that contradicts the one causing the line. If, let us say, you find yourself habitually lifting one eyebrow, thus creating the beginnings of a line across part of your forehead, make a point of lowering that eyebrow as far as it will go from time to time. This will force the skin on your forehead to move in the other direction, and that embryonic line should be minimized.

There are treatments for lines or wrinkles. Some people advocate applying tape to the affected area, forcing the skin into smoothness. I have never done it, so I cannot speak with any great authority about this method, but I do know women who claim they have eliminated budding wrinkles with the tape treatment.

And, of course, you will find dozens of antiwrinkle creams, lotions, and gels in any cosmetics department. You will find women who swear by them, as well as women who swear at them. I am inclined to doubt that anything short of magic will get rid of wrinkles, and I don't believe in magic, so there you are. But you are welcome to try them all.

Of late, people have been talking about the marvelous things aloe vera can do for you. Its advocates claim that it prevents or at least slows down the aging process, and that applications of aloe vera on the skin, or aloe vera taken internally, can make youth linger. My husband is among the aloe vera converts. In fact, he grows the aloe vera plant on the miniranch he maintains at one of the Palm Desert country clubs. He will often go out, pluck a leaf from the plant, slice the leaf with his pocketknife, and rub the white, oily secretion directly on his skin. He claims it works wonders, and I must say his skin looks remarkably good for a man in his eighties.

The aloe vera proponents, who grow almost rabid in their advocacy, claim that aloe vera oil can do almost anything, from stopping a toothache to curing acne. But the oil's main claim to fame is that it helps prevent, or at least slow down, the aging process. I don't use it, because I guess I figure it's too late for me now. If it had come along when I was in my forties I might have figured, well, if this will prevent aging, let's give it a shot. But in my seventies, I am what I am already.

I certainly see nothing wrong in using an aloe vera lotion. I am not so sure about the value of taking this substance internally, but I have not read that it is harmful in any way. Ask your doctor, however, before you try it yourself. My only experience with it has been, as I said, in watching Phil use it, and he just takes it straight—directly from the leaf of the plant to his skin. As far as I know, he doesn't drink it, although, with my husband, you just never can tell.

The one part of my face that I am particularly careful about is my eyes. I believe that when you meet a stranger it is his or her eyes you first notice. Someone has said that the eyes are the mirror of the soul, and that sounds good to me. All I know is that I notice other people's eyes immediately when I meet them, so I suspect they notice mine. That's why I try to keep my eyes as bright and attractive as I possibly can.

Eyes do age. It is not only the skin around them that changes but the eyes themselves. As many of us grow older, our eyes have a tendency to lose their luster; they just look old and tired. But that doesn't have to happen. You can maintain the youthful look of your eyes with a little work and care.

One of the chief enemies of the eyes is the sun. I wear my dark glasses almost constantly when I am outdoors, because I believe direct sunlight has a tendency to dull the sparkle in the eyes over a long period of time.

I also—like virtually everyone else in my age bracket— have to wear prescription glasses for reading. And I wear them, because I have a hunch that making the eyes strain to see is another way to rob them of their natural brilliance. It seems sensible to me that eyes that do not have to work too hard will look better than eyes that do.

Then, too, I try to take particular care of the skin surrounding my eyes. The skin of your eyelids, I was once told, is the thinnest of any part of your body. So I try to keep the area around my eyes clean and moist. When I wash my face, I pay particular attention to that area. And I believe that sufficient sleep is needed for the eyes to retain their luster, too.

While I am not one for heavy makeup, I do use some mascara. My eyelashes are particularly fair, and without mascara I have a tendency to look washed out. So when I am going to be out in public, I do use a bit of mascara.

Some of my friends tell me I don't use enough makeup in general. There have been times when I have been told that I needed more lipstick, or more rouge, or more mascara. But I believe I use enough. I think there is a tendency, among most women, to use too much.

Makeup, for females, has always been fun. Beginning when we were little girls, we loved to make up our faces. I remember trying my mother's big old powder puff when I was just a toddler, and I think every girl goes through that. And we never really lose that love of putting on paint and powder.

But we have to learn, over the years, that a little goes a long way. It's fun—but don't overdo it. Furthermore, I believe that the fairer a person is, the less makeup she should use. Blue-eyed blondes, like me, have to be extra careful, because too much makeup makes us look ridiculous. Women with darker complexions—brown hair, brown eyes—can get away with more makeup; in fact, they look terrible without any makeup at all, whereas us fair ladies can get by with practically none.

I do want to say here, however, that I believe almost every woman should wear at least some makeup. It takes an Ingrid Bergman to get by with none. I used to marvel at her. I would see her at parties, and I don't believe she put a thing on her face other than soap and water, and she always looked ravishing. But there aren't many Ingrid Bergmans running around loose. The rest of us need a little help.

In my case, as I have said, I have these white, white eyelashes, so I must have a bit of mascara, otherwise my face seems to be totally lacking in expression. A little rouge on my cheeks, again to counteract my natural paleness, and a little eye shadow for contrast. And, of course, lipstick. I use a base to cover some tiny red spots on my lips, which I'd rather not have anybody else notice, and then an ordinary lipstick for color. I prefer a light shade, and I wear the same shade day or night. Some women like to use a darker shade at night, but I think I look my best with that same light color at all times.

I imagine my feeling about not wearing much makeup is a natural reaction against all those years of having to wear a great deal. When I appeared on stage and in movies and on TV, I was forced to put an awful lot of glop on my face. And when I walked off the 20th Century–Fox lot for the last time, I got home and washed all of it off my face, and I suppose I overreacted. I said, No more.

So for a while I put nothing on my face in the way of makeup. Literally, nothing. Then I realized that I had to do something, because otherwise I would look like a sheep in a snowstorm—everything pale and wishy-washy. Now I do use some makeup, and I think I have arrived at that happy medium. Not enough makeup that I feel weighted down with it, but enough to highlight my face.

If we are to try to stay young as we grow old, we have to achieve a compromise in the way we make up our faces. What we did as teenagers and young women is no longer practical. Yet we cannot go overboard the other way. This is why I advocate that you see a makeup counselor as you reach new and different plateaus in your life.

Don't try to redesign your makeup yourself. Don't think that you can cover up the signs of aging with a thicker, heavier, gaudier application of makeup. If anything, go easier with it. Have a pro redesign your makeup. Have a pro take a look at your hairstyle and tell you if that, too, needs some work. If you just can't get to consult a professional, pick out a friend you think looks good, and ask her for advice. Or pick up some recent issues of beauty magazines or books. I find it hard to follow the suggestions in those publications, but maybe you'll do better than I.

The main thing is that you get advice from some outside source. We women are the worst judges of our own appearance.

Don't trust your mirror to tell you how you look. Mirror, mirror on the wall is a very prejudiced object. It tells you what you want to see and hear, not what the truth is.

It may say, "Well, dearie, you don't look so bad, for sixty-six. Just put on a little more lipstick, a little brighter eye shadow, a little blonder hair dye, and away you go!"

Don't believe that malarkey. Take that sixty-six-year-old face to a specialist and you'll get another story:

"Well, you're using too much lipstick, tone down your eye shadow, and let your hair go a bit darker."

Don't listen to anybody who might be subjective—husband, lover, children. This is important stuff, so get an honest, objective opinion. You will look your best—and, hence, your most youthful—if you get expert advice and follow it.

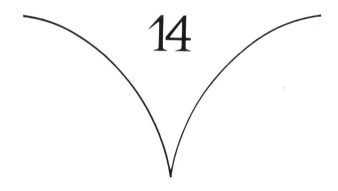

14

W_{hat} about plastic surgery? And, while we're at it, what about cosmetic surgery?

I often wondered what the difference was between these two medical art forms. Actually, I thought they were pretty much synonymous, but there are distinct differences. Cosmetic surgery is performed solely for the sake of the appearance—a nose job is the typical cosmetic surgery. But plastic surgery has as its goal something more than correcting a surface imperfection. Plastic surgery is more serious, more profound. A plastic surgeon works on burn victims, accident victims, people who have been born with major defects in face or form. The plastic surgeon's goal is to make somebody who theretofore was an object of derision or revulsion able to go out into society with an appearance that is as close to normal as is humanly—and medically—possible.

So I am primarily concerned with cosmetic surgery. The pros and cons of plastic surgery are something for some other author to consider.

Actually, very few people, as they grow older and begin to be concerned about aging, need any sort of total plastic surgery. In a few cases age does ravage the face so much that such a procedure is needed, but fortunately those cases are rare. Mostly young elders, if they need any fixing up, require only a little cosmetic surgery, to smooth out a wrinkle here or tighten some sagging flesh there.

In Hollywood tricks to make people look younger than they really are have long been accepted and honorable. It may be only a cinematographer shooting through a piece of gauze to make a lady look softer, but even that can be considered a distant relative of cosmetic surgery. It is a way, after all, of deceiving the eye of the beholder into thinking that a person looks more attractive than he or she actually is. And that, after all, is the purpose of cosmetic surgery.

So I saw that kind of thing all around me in my days as a movie star. When the studio signed a new young man or young woman, they assessed his or her assets and debits. And they did it ruthlessly. The slightest glitch on the body, the merest trifle of an imperfection, would be dealt with harshly.

In many cases the teeth were the first thing to be treated. Virtually every new star had to go to a cosmetic dentist for heavy repair work, fixing gaps in the teeth, or having crowns put over teeth that were crooked. That, too, is cosmetic surgery of a sort. But there were other things. Rita Hayworth, that beauty of beauties, had a hairline the studio moguls felt was too low, so it was fixed surgically. The result was breathtaking.

They desperately wanted to fix Clark Gable's ears, which stuck out at an alarming angle, but he refused. And he made it to the very top with his ears out there like semaphores.

Even if the studio brass did not suggest permanent repairs, they frequently used temporary tricks to get their stars to look their best on screen. Although I never witnessed it myself, we all knew that a favorite weapon of cinematographers and makeup people, working in concert, was the elastic band. When some actors and actresses had a sag here or there, the application of an elastic band at a strategic location pulled the skin back and made it look firm, tight, and young. Rumor had it that Lucille Ball was a prime user of that technique even when she was young, because of some quirk in her facial physiognomy.

Although most Hollywood stars were as close to physically perfect as nature and the law allowed, there were some who had minor flaws. It may have been something as small as a tiny mole on the cheek. Today, I believe, they wouldn't bother with trifles like that, but in my era they wouldn't permit even the slightest blemish to go uncovered. So the makeup men would go to work, and, whatever the imperfection, it would be covered over so the world would never know it existed.

Thus the raw material—the young actor or starlet— would sign a contract, get the full treatment of having teeth fixed, hair restyled, makeup redesigned, and whatever minor imperfections marred his handsomeness or her beauty covered over. In effect, they were all treated to a program of cosmetic surgery. It might not have involved any actual cutting, but the face and form were made over so they looked as good as human hands could make them look.

And there were some who had genuine cosmetic surgery to enhance their attractiveness. Today's movie stars shun such tactics—Barbra Streisand's nose, for example, is her own in all its glory—but in my era she would have been forced to have it surgically altered. It would have been either that or no movie roles.

To me, therefore, cosmetic surgery is a legitimate and accepted form of beauty treatment. I know there are many people who think it is awful for a person—either man or woman—to have cosmetic surgery. But these are the same people who think it is awful for a person—either man or woman—to dye the hair. They have this notion that you mustn't try to fool Mother Nature, that it is wrong to alter your appearance, that doing so is a sin committed for vanity's sake alone.

That is total nonsense. If you follow that reasoning to its logical conclusion, it would also be wrong and sinful to wear clothing. After all, that, too, is altering your appearance with artificial means. I see no difference morally between dyeing your hair or having your nose fixed and wearing a dress.

So if you feel the need for some cosmetic surgery, by all means go for it. If you think you would have a better life if your wrinkles were removed or the bags under your eyes taken away, then have those things done. If you—a man—are going bald and believe your love life or your career would benefit from a hair transplant, then certainly have a hair transplant. If you—a woman—think your chances for the good life would be improved if you had your breasts de-sagged, then do it.

On the other hand, don't do any of these things frivo-lously. They may be trivial, compared with having a brain tumor removed or a triple bypass performed, but they are still surgical procedures. And any time somebody takes a knife to your body, it can be serious.

Even if your treatment does not involve a knife—if you elect a nonsurgical technique, such as face peeling, done with acid applications—it can be a dangerous procedure. An inept practitioner, or a miscalculation, can result in irreparable harm. You must be aware of these potential perils.

A renowned plastic surgeon once told me that he turns away many people who come to him requesting treatment of various sorts. He probably could use the business, but his sense of ethics prevents him from doing the jobs they request.

This is because he believes the procedures they ask for are unnecessary in their cases. He says many women want wrinkles removed or eyelids ironed out and those wrinkles or those eyelids are really not bad looking at all. He cautions these women that the good that could result from such surgery would hardly be worth the trouble, the risk, and—something to be considered—the expense.

Cosmetic surgery, you must realize, is not cheap. And in most cases it is not covered by medical insurance, since the carriers naturally do not consider it necessary to a person's health and well-being. So you have to bear the entire cost yourself, and it is a hefty cost indeed.

The risk is another factor you have to consider very seriously. Any time someone cuts you, there is that element of danger. Cosmetic surgeons, like hairdressers and accountants and cooks, come in all styles—good, bad, and indifferent. And you could be putting yourself, and your face, in the hands of a butcher rather than a surgeon.

I know of a young woman—absolutely gorgeous—who had a modest Hollywood career going. She wasn't a very good actress, but she did reasonably well. Then, as she reached forty or thereabouts, she detected some crow's-feet around her eyes. Everything else about her was still smashing, but she believed that those tiny wrinkles would ruin her career, so she decided to have them removed. But the cosmetic surgeon she went to made a mess of the procedure. The upshot was that this gorgeous woman was badly scarred and today seldom leaves her house. When she does, she wears huge dark glasses and covers the rest of her face with a scarf. Cosmetic surgery, badly performed, ruined her life.

There is another health consideration to be weighed when you are thinking about having some cosmetic surgery performed. And that is your total health picture. Just as you wouldn't have an artificial hip installed if you had a serious heart condition, you shouldn't have cosmetic surgery done if your physical condition could be in any way threatened.

The wonderful comedienne Totie Fields wanted cosmetic surgery done to make her look more attractive. Her doctor warned her that it would be very hard on her physically, because she had a bad heart. Apparently, she felt it was worth the risk, so she had the work done. And, because of it, she died. As her physician had feared, it was too much for her heart to take.

Surgery, no matter how minor it may appear, is still a strain on the system. So before you arrange to have any cosmetic surgery done, be sure to see your personal doctor, tell him or her what you are contemplating, and ask if it is safe for you to go ahead with your plans. If your doctor says no, it is too risky given your total health picture, then don't do it. After all, the way you look is hardly a matter of life and death. But if your physician gives you the green light, and you believe the procedure will give you a better life, and if you can afford it without stress or strain on the budget, then by all means do it. Don't let people tout you off it by saying that it goes against nature or that if God wanted you to have fewer wrinkles He would have made you that way. Answer those arguments with the unbeatable comeback "If God wanted me to wear clothes, He would have had them on me when I was born."

The whole point of anything you do to yourself—from putting lipstick on your lips to having a cosmetic surgery done—is to make you feel better within yourself. The trick in mastering life is to be confident in who you are and what you are. I know that's true because, as I have said, I was never very confident about myself in my early years. I was so unsure of myself that I was convinced that one morning I would wake up and find that all this about being a movie star had been a dream. I really wasn't a movie star at all, just a kid from New York struggling to make it in the chorus line. I needed all the help in the confidence department that I could get. Some of it came from cosmetics—as I told you in Chapter 13, I had learned, from makeup men, how to make the most of what I had, and cosmetics helped in that area.

So you put on a front. You may be quaking and insecure inside, but if you put on that brave front, nobody knows how your insides are quaking. Whatever helps you with that front is to the good. If you know you look good—as good as you possibly can—then you have taken a giant step from being insecure to being positive and self-possessed. So whatever helps you feel good about yourself—from hair dye to cosmetic surgery—is a step in the right direction.

We all go through life trying to project an image of strength and self-confidence. I used to get a kick out of the fact that, no matter how unsure of myself I was, people would come up to me and say, "Alice, I admire you so much because you are always so positive." That happened to me so often; I would be shivering in my boots and they would say I was so positive.

That's what having confidence in the way you look can do for you. It can make you project an image of assuredness, even while you feel you are nothing very much. Whatever you can do to your outside to give you that appearance of self-confidence on the inside is beneficial. Which is why I applaud those who feel that cosmetic surgery is something they need. If it goes even a small way toward improving a person's self-image, then it is a very good thing.

Most of us get kicked around a lot in our lifetimes. Life is a series of rejections, and rejections are tough to take. In my profession—the acting business—rejection becomes a close personal friend. You get rejected so often you feel like you are living in a revolving door. You turn the other cheek so often you need a neck with a built-in ratchet.

So we all need whatever added help we can get, and if it

comes out of a can of hair dye or from the ministrations of a cosmetic surgeon, what difference does it make? As long as it makes you feel better about yourself, and as long as it can't hurt you, it's a positive step.

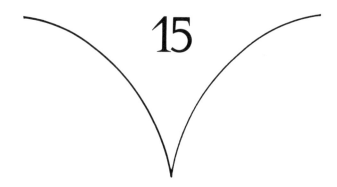

15

In the last chapter I talked about how your eyes are what make the strongest impression on people you meet. There are those who would dispute this statement. There are those who believe that what people first notice about you is not your eyes, or even your face, but what you wear. They claim, with a certain logic, that since your clothing takes up at least 90 percent of your total surface, it is naturally what people first notice when they meet you.

I believe it is a combination of elements that people first notice—the sum of all the parts. It isn't just the face and it isn't just the clothing, it is everything.

In his book, *Dressing to Win,* fashion expert Robert Pante says this:

Think of your own reaction when you meet someone for the first time. What is the first thing you are aware of?

Is it the face? The figure? The clothing? The look in the eyes? The way the hair is combed? The jewelry? The shine on the shoes?

Probably it is not any one single thing, but the total combined effect of all of them. All those elements work together to create one overall picture. What we notice is the *total* appearance, the sum of all the parts.

I have looked better in some pictures than in others because of the costumes I was required to wear. Audiences have the notion that the stars pick out their wardrobes, but this is rarely true. You wear what you are told to wear, just as you say the words you are told to say and move where you are told to move. At least in my time that's the way it was. I don't know about today.

In *Every Night at Eight* I was forced to wear a series of fussy outfits—sequins, furs, velvets, lace—that made me look foolish. The costumes I was squeezed into in *Sing, Baby, Sing* were dismissed by one reviewer as "atrocious," and I think he was kind. In *Wake Up and Live* I wore a caricature of a man's suit with extremely wide lapels, and one reviewer called the costumes in that film "a nightmare of bad taste."

On the other hand, in *You're a Sweetheart* the designer gave me costumes that were simple and elegant, mostly in basic black or not-so-basic silver. *Tin Pan Alley* was famous for the authenticity and stylishness of its pre–World War I costumes, and I enjoyed wearing them—even the hobble skirts.

Mostly, I was supposed to look glamorous. But in *Tail Spin,* a film about aviation, I wore almost nothing but flying suits. And I like to think I looked like an authentic aviator. I created the impression of an aviator. What I wore in films was generally designed to create an impression. That is true in real life, too—what we wear creates a vivid impression in the eyes of the people we meet. And that, I believe, makes good sense. Our wardrobe obviously contributes a great deal to that "one overall picture" Pante talks about. So let us now consider wardrobe.

High fashion is for the young primarily. Dress designers, when they create their new styles, usually do not have us young elders in mind. They design for women in their twenties, thirties, and forties, who are generally the fashion leaders. It is, therefore, up to us ourselves to forge fashions for our age-group, our use. And the first thing we must realize is that it isn't easy for us to look smart yet not foolish.

We can't wear what our daughters and granddaughters are wearing. Nothing looks as ridiculous as a woman in her sixties thinking she can wear current fad fashions. In the days of the flower children, some women in their sixties and beyond tried to keep in step with that noble movement and dress like flower children. They looked more like last year's bouquets. Flower children styles, as their name implies, were exclusively for the young. Nobody said anything about flower women. So don't think you can copy the styles of the very young. Let the very young have them. They are their property.

On the other hand, I don't want you to dress as some other women do. When they reach their fiftieth birthday, they throw away everything in their closets that isn't black, brown, or gray. Gone is everything with any color, any dash, any style. They become frumps and dress frumpishly from then on, because they apparently believe that over fifty means over the hill.

There is a happy medium.

I like color. I often wear pink. Maybe bright green. And

other colors. Black is fine, too; in fact, I think I look good in black, because it contrasts nicely with my fair coloring. But I really prefer bright colors.

As for the styling of clothes for our age-group, I believe anything goes—within reason. I think the classic styles are the best. Ever since I began my film career, I have preferred to dress in tailored clothes, created along classic lines. I never have liked the fussy things, the dresses with buttons and bows and other folderol. I have a large wardrobe of tailored suits, tailored blouses and shirts, and slack suits.

In fact, I am usually in a slack suit. Of course, you have to keep in pretty good shape to wear a slack suit. Nothing looks worse than a large, overweight lady stuffed into a slack suit designed with a slender lady in mind. If you like to wear slack suits, you must keep yourself in shape.

The same thing applies to shorts. I like to wear shorts in the extreme hot weather we often get in the Coachella Valley, and fortunately my legs are still good. But you women with hefty bottoms and fat legs, please do not wear shorts, no matter how comfortable they are. They just look terrible on you if you are too large in those areas.

The thing about tailored, classic outfits is that women of all ages can wear them. And, of course, they are never out of style, so you can wear them year after year. Once in a while you may have to raise or lower the hem an inch or so, but otherwise they stay comfortably in style continuously. That tailored look flatters most women, I believe, and it is particularly flattering for young elders. It looks stylish without looking too fancy. There is an elegance to that look that is consistent with our age-group. Being a young elder brings with it an automatic elegance—the elegance of maturity—and the tailored look carries out that theme perfectly.

At our age there are some things we should studiously avoid, because of certain quirks in our appearance brought on by the years. Our necks, shoulders, and arms are no longer as firm as they once were, so we should steer clear of low-cut dresses, or any type of sleeveless garments or scoop neck-lines. I know I can't wear a sleeveless dress anymore. It may be comfortable, but I don't think I look good in it. So I have removed all sleeveless dresses and blouses from my closet.

You have to be able to assess your own appearance ruth-lessly this way. If you have assets, show them. If you have debits, don't. You should know what you have and what you don't have by this time, so act accordingly.

One of the things many of us no longer have is a slim, trim, and snazzy figure. While my own is still in reasonably good condition, I am only too aware that there are a lot of pudgy people out there. So while we are in the business of ruthlessly assessing our appearance, let's not forget the over-all look we present to people—our figures.

If your figure is something less that perfect, don't wear clothing that calls attention to it. I remember once going to see a movie in which a famous actress took off her clothes, and there wasn't much left after the clothes were off—she was pretty scrawny. And Phil growled, in his inimitable growl, "If you don't got it, don't flaunt it!" So if you no longer have a neat figure, you should attempt to camouflage it as best you can. Fortunately, there are ways of doing just that.

Loose, flowing garments are the best camouflage. Things such as caftans and muumuus, capes and other outfits that are attractive but do not hug the body are ideal. They hide the shape within while giving the outward appearance of good style.

If your legs have thickened over the years, wear slacks most of the time. Nobody knows, when you're wearing slacks, if your legs are thick or as beautiful as Betty Grable's were. Whatever you do, don't fall prey to current fashion and wear a miniskirt (if that's current this second). Only kids or ladies with incredibly beautiful legs should wear minis, or any style that calls attention to their legs. Actually, it is not only thick or terribly thin legs that look terrible in short skirts. Bony knees are another debit in the leg department, and I have seen so many women walking around in minis with their bony knees rattling in the breeze.

Be brutal in your self-assessment. If your body is not what it used to be—or perhaps it never was what you thought it used to be—then by all means select clothing that covers it up as much as possible. Fashions today are forgiving; by that I mean you can find clothing that forgives you your faults by covering them up very nicely and smartly.

There are many men, I know, who are still knocked for a loop by a shapely ankle. A trim ankle, peeking out from beneath a midcalf-length skirt, seems to give promise of great things above. So no matter how thick your legs or how bony your knees, chances are your ankles are still ready for attraction. Take advantage of that, wear those midcalf-length skirts, and send your ankles out to do the job that the rest of your legs can't do anymore.

All of the above can apply to men as well as women. If you have developed a paunch, a potbelly, gone flabby around your middle, then you shouldn't wear tight-fitting clothes. Wear loose shirts and sweaters. Don't wear bikini-bottom bathing trunks, because a man looks foolish and unattractive with all that flesh hanging over his swim trunks. Wear looser, boxer-style trunks to the beach; you may not look like Sylvester Stallone or Hulk Hogan, but you won't look like a baby blimp either.

Color is a very important consideration in choosing your wardrobe. The importance of that fact was brought home to me strongly in 1939, when I did a film called *Hollywood Cavalcade*. That was my first Technicolor movie. Until then the only thing the camera could distinguish was shades of black, white, and gray. But suddenly I had to become conscious of what colors were best for me.

Some people simply do not look good in certain colors,

and others do. It has a great deal, of course, to do with your own natural coloring—but not everything. There are certain intangibles present, so you cannot say that just because you are a brunette you will look good in red. Most brunettes do, but some simply don't.

You have to analyze your own color preferences very closely. Color charts are a good way to begin if you have doubts. Now I personally have never used one, because the studio wardrobe people, who were the tops in their trade, picked out my clothing for me when I was at Fox, and I could see what looked good on me and what didn't. But most people do not have the good fortune to have the world's leading clothing experts dressing them. For these people, a color chart consultation is a wise investment. You'll find color charts at the top department and specialty stores, where experts will take you in hand and show you which colors and color combinations are best for you.

Being well dressed is often as simple as doing things like picking out garments that camouflage your weaknesses and feature colors that flatter you. It is primarily a matter of using your good features and minimizing your bad. I'm considered well dressed, but I wouldn't be if I wore things that showed me to a disadvantage.

At the studio I had a wardrobe woman, Ollie Hughes, who was with me for many years. She had been assigned to me at first and got to know me and my clothing so well that she was a great comfort to me. She knew all my clothing quirks, knew when I wanted to put my shoes on and when I wanted to take them off (which is important when you're on your feet all day), and took care of all my wardrobe needs. I never missed being a movie star, but I must confess there are days when I wish I had Ollie, my personal wardrobe gal, around to help me.

I like to wear hats. I think they look good on me, and I enjoy the feeling of having a hat on my head. Besides, the broad-brimmed ones I favor serve a utilitarian purpose. They shade my eyes from the sun, which can be pretty glaring in the desert area where I live. Then, too, since I swim so much, my hair is usually a mess, and a hat is a great way of covering up that mess.

Hats have been a part of my personal style for many years now. The studio wardrobe people put me in hats frequently in films—everything from country bonnets to sailor hats—and I think those wardrobe people were very clever about making us actors and actresses look our best. I have always felt that they must have put me in hats for some reason, so I keep on wearing hats. And I like what hats do for me.

Shoes are important, too. As we get older, we have to understand that high heels must go. That's part of the business about being careful about falling, because our bones are getting more brittle all the time. High heels are a threat at any age—when you wear them, your balance is precarious—but as we get older that threat becomes more and more serious. Besides, I believe high heels are another style that belongs to the younger generation. I hate the phrase "sensible shoes," because it conjures up a picture of heavy black clodhoppers, but we really do have to wear sensible shoes as we get older. That doesn't mean they have to be those clodhoppers, though.

Shoes can be sensible and attractive. As more and more women reach the young-elder plateau, shoe manufacturers are becoming more and more conscious of this growing market. So they are creating styles in flat-heeled shoes that are very lovely.

I wear very low heels on almost all my shoes. I still have a few pairs of party shoes with a slightly higher heel, but nothing that would even remotely be considered a genuine high heel. By far, most of my shoes are ones with low heels. I have walking shoes, and, of course, they have only the slightest heel. When I travel I wear low-heeled shoes because

I have to do a lot of traipsing through airports, and I don't want to risk another accident of tripping and falling. And on the plane itself I like to slip my shoes on and off easily.

I know there are a lot of women, even older than I am, who still cling to their high heels. This is, I believe, a vanity trip. They just cannot give up those high heels, which they apparently equate with youth. As long as they can wear their high heels, they believe they are still young and beautiful. But they are also risking serious injury.

What about jewelry as we get older? The same rules apply, I believe. The wild, gaudy jewelry of youth is inappropriate for us young elders. We look foolish if we are obviously in our sixties or seventies and sporting costume jewelry designed with teenagers in mind. But, again, that doesn't mean we should go around as unadorned as plucked chickens.

Phil always says he's a lucky man, because jewelry has never meant very much to me. There are some women, as we all know, who worship jewelry so much that everything their husbands or boyfriends earn goes into diamonds, rubies, and sapphires. And then most of the time they are so afraid of their precious gems being stolen that they keep them in safe deposit vaults in their banks. They visit their jewels but never get a chance to wear them. Phil has never particularly liked jewelry either. Even in our courting days his gifts were not in the jewelry department. So I just never got in the habit of acquiring expensive jewelry, and I must say it's never meant very much in my life.

This may also have something to do with the fact that, when I was in pictures, I frequently wore very ritzy jewels. On several occasions the studio borrowed jewelry from one of the high-class stores for me to wear, and there were armed guards around the studio while I wore necklaces and bracelets and earrings that were bursting with carats. I had more diamonds than One-a-Day has vitamin pills. I once even had jewel-studded stockings; for a number in *On the Avenue,* I wore these stockings with jewels sewed onto them, which were pretty snazzy. Although I realized these fancy jewels were beautiful, I never was consumed with envy. At the end of each day's shooting, I gave them all back—even the stockings—without a second thought.

I have some things I enjoy. I do like gold chains, and I have quite a few in different weights and lengths. I like what has come to be known as the Chanel look in jewelry—a gold chain and a pair of simple gold earrings. To me, that is a very elegant look—neat but hardly gaudy. And I think elegance is what we should strive for in our young-elder years. Whereas once our goal might have been to be exciting and possibly even a touch flashy, now I believe the goal should be quiet, understated elegance.

People often ask me if I got to keep any of the beautiful costumes I wore in films. As a rule, no actor or actress gets to keep what is worn before the camera. Those things go back into the wardrobe department and usually are worn again, with some alterations, by other actors and actresses in other films.

Many of the things I wore in films would have been no use to me even if they had been given to me. That's because so many of my films were period pieces. In movies such as *Lillian Russell, In Old Chicago,* and *Hello, Frisco, Hello,* I was decked out in costumes that were authentic copies of fashions of the last century. They were fun to wear, but what good would they do me in the twentieth century? (Of course, today's kids would have a ball with them, snipping here and slicing there and making something they would wear anywhere, even to school.)

In those days Hollywood wardrobe departments didn't stint on anything. I understand that they are not as careful about things today, but when I was at the peak of my career, the wardrobe people were justifiably proud of their work.

Why, even the corsets and other undergarments they provided us with were lovely.

Everything was handmade. We used to think it was a pity the audience never got to see those undergarments, because they were things of remarkable beauty. I remember one corset I wore in *Lillian Russell* that was trimmed in the finest lace and really was a work of art. But nobody ever saw it except me and the wardrobe department.

Still, it made me feel special, and perhaps that was the whole point. Maybe it was psychological, so that we actors would believe ourselves to be larger than life and that would come across on the screen. Acting, you know, is all make-believe, and the more you believe you are the person you're portraying, the better your portrayal. So perhaps having all those fancy, handmade undergarments helped me to believe that I really was, say, Lillian Russell, and that might have made my characterization more believable.

My life then was, in retrospect, almost like being part of a real fairy tale. It wasn't only the lace-trimmed corsets but the whole business of being a star. They even had music on the set, as we waited for the lights and the cameras and all the equipment to be made ready for the next shot. It all contributed to the feeling that you were part of a fantasy, that this wasn't reality at all but some unbelievable world into which you had stumbled and in which you really didn't belong.

I mean, every once in a while I would look in the mirror and say to myself, "Who do you think you are kidding, Alice? All of this isn't for you, it's for somebody else. Now, take off that fancy corset and go back to the West Fifties, where you belong." But it *was* for me, and I *did* belong there. I am digressing, however, from the subject of this chapter, which is the fashions appropriate for young elders.

If you are like I am, you love clothes. Most women do. These days I am mad about clothes. I love beautiful things—

Chanel clothes and Adolfo suits, things by Bill Blass and David Hayes. I must admit that I love expensive clothing. I enjoy shopping in New York, and one of my dreams is to get to the showings in Paris some year.

Just because we women like good clothing doesn't mean that we have to go out and spend our last nickel on a fancy dress, but it does mean that we like to look our best every hour of every day. I confess that I love nice clothes. And I have what I consider a pretty nifty wardrobe. Every time Phil says anything about my spending so much on clothes, I tell him it is all the fault of the cleaners. It's nice to have a convenient scapegoat. I blame the Russians when the weather is bad, and I blame the cleaners for the fact that I have so many clothes.

There is, I believe, some truth in my assertion that it is the cleaners' fault. (I am not so sure about the Russians and the weather, although who knows?) But it does seem to me that the cleaners are increasingly rough on clothing these days, and so often I get a garment back from the cleaners that is damaged so badly I can't wear it again. And so, naturally, I have to go out and get two new ones to replace it. Or I wear something once and then send it to be cleaned and it comes back so tight I can't get into it—and I haven't gained that much. Then, of course, I have to get two others to replace that one.

My closets bulge with good clothing, and I think that's only fair and just. After all, I feel I need all the help I can get. I am big with slack suits. I have suits, skirts, blouses, shorts, and a lot of swimwear. Not too many dresses, although I am able to get togged out when the occasion arises and look pretty good. Like most women, I have a few of what I call my "knock 'em dead" dresses, things that I know will make a very big impression on any crowd.

But with everything I own I keep in mind who I am and how old I am. My daughters and granddaughters can wear the newer styles, the fad fashions. I would look silly in them. So I wear things that are right for my age. I don't mean that I wear anything frumpy or dowdy, because I don't. Everything I have is stylish and elegant, but it is not high fashion.

I don't read *Vogue* and run out and buy something with feathers because feathers are all the rage in Paris this season. I buy something this year that I am pretty sure will look just as good next year and probably five years from now, too.

If you want to Grow Older but Stay Young, be careful about your clothing. Don't wear something that will make people turn around and snicker at you after you pass by. Wear your age, which doesn't mean stark old-lady clothes, but does mean classically simple lines. Strive for elegance, not gaudiness.

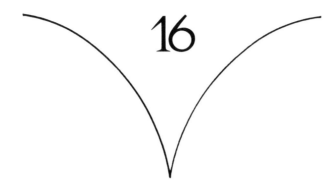

16

You are starting to get old when you read the obituary page before you read the front page in your daily newspaper. But you are *really* starting to get old when most of the obits on that page report the deaths of people younger than you.

So many of my old friends are gone. I haven't much left in the way of family—my parents, my two brothers are gone. And so many of the people I worked with in my movie career have passed away, too—Tyrone Power, Betty Grable, George Raft, Patsy Kelly, Jack Oakie, Jack Haley, Dick Powell, Jimmy Durante, Al Jolson, and the list goes on. Sometimes I think that Don Ameche and I are the only ones still around from Hollywood's golden years.

It is that fact—the feeling that we are leftovers—that makes so many of us young elders fall into pits of depression.

The Public Health Service of the U.S. Department of Health and Human Services estimates that as many as 30 percent of people over sixty-five suffer from depression, often so severe they require treatment. And—another grim statistic—people over the age of fifty-five account for almost one-third of all suicides in America.

Yet not enough attention and money are given to the mental needs of young elders. I suppose this is primarily because for centuries people have mistakenly believed that it is the normal thing to become depressed as we grow older. So why bother to do anything about it?

But, of course, that simply isn't true. Depression isn't something that automatically happens to you when you pass your sixty-fifth birthday. It is not a must. It is not a given.

First, what is meant by depression, exactly?

The National Institute of Mental Health lists the following symptoms of classic depression:

1. A persistent sad, anxious, or empty mood.
2. Feelings of hopelessness and/or pessimism.
3. Feelings of guilt, helplessness, and worthlessness.
4. A loss of interest in pleasure, in daily activities, in sex.
5. Poor sleeping habits (either lack of sleep or over-sleeping).
6. Poor eating habits (either malnutrition or obesity).
7. Loss of energy and a constant feeling of fatigue.
8. Restlessness and irritability.
9. Contemplation of suicide and preoccupation with thoughts of death.
10. Difficulty in remembering, in concentrating, and the inability to reach a decision.

There are several reasons why people become depressed. One of the main ones is the prospect of facing an old age without adequate financial resources. Social Security has gone a long way toward alleviating that fear, but it hasn't eliminated it. In many cases Social Security is still inadequate. It really doesn't make any difference how much money you have, you can still worry about whether you will have enough when you grow too old to earn more.

I learned a valuable lesson about money early in my career. When I was starting out at 20th Century–Fox, the great humorist and actor Will Rogers was still at the studio. Although I never had a chance to work with him, I did meet him, and we ate lunch together quite a few times in the studio commissary. He was notorious for being tight with a buck, and he once talked about his philosophy about money. "Let me tell you, young lady," he said to me, "if you have so much money that you have to sit up all night worrying about it, then the Hell with it. I never worry about money." He just hung on to it, and they used to say that Will had the first dime he ever made. That, of course, is a form of worrying about it, and Will Rogers was like everybody else—he was concerned about his old age. Unfortunately, he never lived to cash in on his frugality.

Worrying about our financial future is a very normal thing to do. None of us wants to be poor when we are no longer able to take care of ourselves. But, tragically, there are millions of people who live at or below the poverty level in their old age. And none of us wants to be dependent on children or grandchildren at that point in our lives either. We all would like to be self-sufficient, able to pay our bills, able to live with dignity and some measure of comfort and security.

It is too late to do much about this problem when you are in your sixties or seventies. Obviously, this is something you should prepare for when you are young and strong, when your earning power is at its peak. Today, thanks to IRAs and other financial niceties in addition to Social Security, it is possible for almost everyone to set aside enough money to guarantee a secure tomorrow. Almost—but not quite everyone yet.

The other major source of depression for young elders is the prospect of loneliness. So many people, surrounded by friends and family for all their lives, wake up one dreadful morning to find themselves totally alone. Their friends have died. Their relatives have died or moved to distant cities or, in the worst possible scenario, no longer want to be bothered with them. So they find themselves sitting in rooms somewhere, or living in the same old houses, and there is nobody to talk to, nobody who gives a damn whether they live or die, nobody period. It is enough to depress anybody.

Unlike the financial problem, however, the problem of loneliness can be dealt with, and conquered. If you find yourself in this situation, you have to make an effort yourself. You cannot just sit in that room, or rattle around in that house, and spend the rest of your life feeling sorry for yourself. Nobody is going to help you unless you begin by trying to help yourself.

Get out and do something.

Do some volunteer work at a nearby hospital or children's home or museum, as I discussed in Chapter 10.

Get a part-time job, even if it is something as menial as delivering pizzas or being a cashier in a supermarket.

Join a club or some sort of organization. Have you always wanted to act? Join your local little theater; they are always short of people to play the older, character roles in plays. And those roles, actors know, are usually the meatiest ones.

Take part in your church's activities.

Enroll in an extension course at your local college or high school, even if it means taking a subject in which you don't have much interest. At least it will bring you into contact with other people, and that will mean the end of your loneliness. And, after all, that's the name of this particular game.

There are dozens of ways you can meet people, in many cases people who are in the same boat you are. In many cities you will find agencies that bring lonely people together to share living quarters. Sometimes these agencies arrange for private homes to be made available to three or four people who are at loose ends. Together they can afford such a house, and they share the expenses, the work, and the pleasure of having companionship. These agencies also try to find room-mates for people who are alone.

If you are still healthy, you might consider taking a job as a companion for some elderly person who can no longer take care of himself or herself. Often these people need assistance but cannot afford to hire a full-time person. There are agencies in this area as well. Such arrangements kill two cases of loneliness with one generous deed.

Another way of ending loneliness and simultaneously feeling useful is through one of the many surrogate grandparent programs that are becoming popular in many cities. These groups bring together children who have no grandparents or whose grandparents live in distant cities and young elders who similarly have no grandchildren or none close by. The surrogate grandparents visit their substitute grandchildren once or twice a week and do the things grandparents usually do with their grandchildren—they spoil them outrageously. It is fun for everybody, the spoilers and the spoiled alike.

Another recent development is the "granny flat." This idea began in Australia, made its way to Canada, and has recently begun to have an impact in the United States. The idea is to build a small, inexpensive building—just a little living room, tiny bedroom, and a kitchen and bath—and place it near the home of family members. Thus, the grannies or the grandpas, or both, have privacy yet are close to their loved ones. In Australia and Canada the government pays the cost of putting the building on the lot and then, when it is no longer needed, moves it somewhere else, where another family can use it.

So there are many ways in which you, as a young elder, can find a place of your own and people who will ease that terrible feeling of being all alone.

If all human resources fail you and loneliness is still on your mind, give serious thought to acquiring a pet. A dog, a cat, a bird, even some tropical fish can ease that lonely feeling considerably. The Ralston Purina people (they make pet food, so they have an ax to grind, of course) have sponsored a program they call Pets for People, and they tell me they have been responsible for placing more than fifteen thousand pets with elderly, lonely people. They claim it's a big help. I think they are probably right; I know I can never be lonely as long as I have my dogs with me.

If your depression becomes severe, you should consult your doctor. There are prescription drugs that do wonders for alleviating depression. Your physician may suggest you talk to a psychiatrist. Don't let that word scare you, because it doesn't mean you are crazy. A psychiatrist is merely a specialist in problems affecting the mental attitude, and he or she has ways of dealing with conditions such as depression.

It is no fun to be depressed. It isn't easy to overcome, but it is not impossible to overcome either. You must first discover what is the root of that depression, and then do something to change the conditions that brought it on. If it is loneliness, get out and get busy and find some new friends. If it is money, that is a tougher nut to crack, but you can do it—find ways to cut your expenses, perhaps by sharing living quarters with someone else or by moving to a less expensive home or apartment or room. Perhaps you can get some kind of part-time job to increase your income; or, if that is not possible, see if some sort of government money is coming to you.

The first place to go to find remedies for whatever is depressing you is your local social service agency. The workers there are trained and, by and large, proficient. They know the laws, they know the possibilities, they know the problems and will have several solutions to offer you.

Many people still cling to that noble but outdated notion that it is wrong to seek charity. In the first place, don't think of things like Social Security and food stamps as charity; in most cases you are simply getting back in them money you have paid out previously in the form of taxes or deductions from your paycheck. People who refuse such government aid are putting their pride before their common sense. Refusing charity might have been brave and upright in pioneer days, but it no longer makes sense.

Another source of depression is something new in our society, but it should be considered. It is the fact that we young elders are, more and more, being discriminated against. The American Association of Retired Persons calls this "ageism," which is like racism, only directed at people solely because of how old they are. What makes the fact of this discrimination so absurd is that there are more and more of us. We may be a minority today—only one in four Americans is over fifty now—but within a short while we will be the majority of our population.

But nowadays there are so many signs of such discrimination around. There are the stereotypes on television and in the movies showing older people as crotchety or addle brained or in their second childhood. There is the widely held view that when you get old you should be bundled off to a nursing home, whereas in reality more than two-thirds of all America's elderly people live by themselves and flourish very well independently. And in many industries there is still the idea that people over sixty-five can no longer work, so they are forced to retire.

We who are in our sixties, seventies, and eighties look out at the world and see these signs of discrimination and wonder why. I know I myself often see signs of it, yet I feel young—I feel as good as I ever did—and I don't believe there is anything I can't handle, except maybe bronco busting.

The fact that people tend to lump all of us young elders in the same pot, and label that pot "Old Fogies," is very depressing to me. I am not an old fogy, and I never will be. I believe that half the battle against depression is keeping the belief that you are still a vital and very alive individual. What matters most to me is how I feel on the inside, and Alice Faye still feels like a girl.

I realize I am more fortunate than many people in those two key factors—finances and friends. I am not rich, but I will never have to worry about keeping a roof over my head and food on my table. And, even though many of my best friends have died, I still have others. Then, of course, I have my husband and my two daughters and my grandchildren, so I am not lonely.

There is one other solution to the question of loneliness that I must mention. And that is the possibility of romance when you are a young elder. So many of us are widows. I remember seeing a statistic that for every fifty men over the age of sixty-five there are one hundred women in that age bracket. Even those fifty men are, by and large, widowers. So there are a lot of single people around, men and women alike.

Why shouldn't they get together? Life is so much better if it is a shared experience. I know when I travel by myself I often see something marvelous, and I want to turn to Phil and say, "Look at that—isn't that beautiful?" But he isn't there, so I can't say, "Look at that—isn't that beautiful?" to anybody but myself. And that's no fun. We all enjoy companionship, having someone to share experiences with. More and more we are coming around to the realization that there is nothing wrong with two people over sixty-five falling in love and sharing the rest of their lives.

There may be sex involved in that relationship or there may only be companionship. There may be marriage, or maybe the couple will just decide to live together. It could be simpler that way, and I think today's society no longer requires a marriage license to make a relationship binding.

It is possible for people to meet in many different settings. Church has always been a great spot for making friends, of all sorts. If you work or join a club or go to a class, you find many opportunities for making new friends, of both sexes.

If you have lost your husband, or your wife, I do not mean to suggest that you must rush out and form a liaison with the first person of the opposite sex who gives you the time of day. But don't just curl up in a ball and wither away. Your late mate would probably want you to be happy, and he or she would know that you don't want to be all alone for the rest of your life. So it is not disloyal to him or her if you begin to see a particular person and, eventually, if you begin a relationship with that person. It is a very natural thing to do.

Depression, then, is a state of mind that can affect anyone at any time. But it is most common in our age-group because the things that cause depression—worry about concerns such as money and loneliness and health—can come to a head in the young-elder years. But each of these worries can be overcome. This chapter has looked at how the money problem and loneliness can be conquered. And we have talked in earlier chapters about ways of preserving your health. All the primary causes of depression can be dealt with, and we can and should live out our lives in mental serenity.

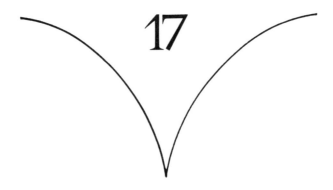

17

I have mentioned often in this book the fact that I recognize how lucky I am in several ways. I have been fortunate in the fact that I am financially secure. I was fortunate in the family I happened to be born into, a family blessed with good genes that contribute greatly toward the way I look—my coloring, my figure—and my health.

And I had some lucky breaks in my career as well. One of my best roles was in the big epic *In Old Chicago,* which was taken from Niven Busch's novel called *We, the O'Learys,* which climaxed with the big 1871 Chicago fire. The part I played had been written with Jean Harlow in mind. But when Jean died, there was an opening. The director, Henry King, asked for me. And I got that plum part.

That's the way the cookie crumbles in Hollywood. One person's tragedy turned out to be my good fortune. When I decided to retire, years later, that decision turned out to be a lucky break for another girl—Ginger Rogers. The studio had bought *Roxie Hart* with me in mind, but after I quit there was one of those openings, and Ginger Rogers stepped in and filled it. It turned out to be one of the best things she ever did. It would have been a fun part for me, too, but I think I made the right decision.

Lucky breaks are part of life's menu for all of us. And among them are the dual questions of friends and family, two items that are of vital importance to our spiritual well-being.

I have had a marriage that has worked and is still working, with a husband—Phil Harris, of course—who is still alive and ticking and still an integral part of my life. And I have two terrific daughters and four grandchildren. And I have had many good friends down through the years. Some have passed away—in fact, my best friend has left me—but I have others.

It seems to me that having family and friends close by who are ready, willing, and able to help you when you need help is a terribly important part of Growing Older but Staying Young. What was that old Dean Martin song? "Everybody Loves Somebody Sometime." If we are to stay young, we must have help from time to time, even if it is only a shoulder to lean on and a pair of ears to tell your troubles to. You can't do it alone. Being alone is an unnatural state, which is why there are so few happy hermits.

I do believe, however, that we all need some privacy, some moments to be by ourselves. There are couples, I realize, who spend every waking moment together and then sleep together, too. Good for them. But for me, and for Phil, too, there are times when we want to get away and just be alone.

Henry David Thoreau, who spent those productive seasons alone on the shores of Walden Pond, once wrote: "I never found the companion that was so companionable as solitude."

But just as I believe in a balanced diet, I believe in balanced companionship—sometimes I need to be with people, sometimes (to echo that phrase Garbo never really said), I want to be alone.

The thing is, basically, that it is nice to have a man around the house—when I need and want him. And it is nice to have children and grandchildren handy—when I feel the urge to be motherly and grandmotherly. And it is nice to have friends I can call, and call on—when I desire friendship. But it is equally nice to be able to go off by myself, with maybe a dog or two or maybe not even them, and just meditate or daydream or have a grand old time doing absolutely nothing.

I am fortunate, again, in that Phil feels the same way. He doesn't always want me fussing over him, or hanging on to his every joke. Sometimes he, too, wants a dash of solitude, a pinch of peace and quiet.

People often ask me the secret of our long, successful marriage. Hollywood, of course, has the reputation for producing marriages that generally last ten minutes or so. But I believe there are just as many long-lived marriages in Hollywood as there are in Peoria—look at how long people such as John Forsythe, Ricardo Montalban, Claudette Colbert, and many others have been married.

Phil and I were married on May 12, 1941. Since that was seven months before Pearl Harbor, it is almost ancient history. We have been married for forty-nine years now, and, assuming the gods are with us, we look forward to celebrating our golden wedding anniversary in 1991, which is just around the calendar.

Anyhow, when people ask me the secret of a long marriage, I say that, first and foremost, luck plays a big part. Then good health—you can't have a long marriage if one of the two participants dies. And third, and maybe most important, we give each other some elbowroom. He does his thing; I do my thing. We don't lean on each other constantly. We are there, if one of us needs a helping hand or a broad shoulder, but there is plenty of room for individual freedom. I recognize that may not be what everybody wants in a marriage. It works for us, but it might not work for people who think a marriage, by definition, means that the two halves combine to make one individual whole, and that husband and wife must be together constantly and forevermore.

Phil and I had met, casually, once or twice, but nothing came of it. We were both married to other people at the time of those early, brief encounters. For many years Jack Oakie called himself our Dan Cupid, claiming to have been the one who introduced us. It is possible that he was right about that, because one night while I was shooting a movie called *That Night in Rio,* I was dancing at the old Charlie Foy's Supper Club when Oakie danced by and dragged me over to introduce me to his old buddy Phil Harris. Both Phil and I think we may have met each other at an earlier date, but maybe not. It is of no earth-shattering significance. At any rate, Oakie did introduce us, but nothing happened for a while.

Some time later, by coincidence, Phil and I were both living in Encino, which is in the San Fernando Valley above Los Angeles. And, by another coincidence, we both owned Doberman pinschers at the time. A third coincidence was that by then we were both single again.

In the morning I would let my dog out early. I had to get up to be at the studio in time to have my hair and makeup done, and I figured it was OK to let my dog loose at that hour, so he could run around for a while. Who would be up at four in the morning? But Phil was working, too, and he had let his Doberman out, too, and the two dogs met on the street and got into a terrible fight. So Mr. Harris called me up and yelled at me and told me what I could do with my dog, and I told him what he could do with his dog. It was quite a lovely argument, because we both have a way with words.

We met to discuss it some more. And Phil suggested we continue the discussion over dinner. We did have dinner, and I don't think we mentioned Doberman pinschers once. And so we began dating, and that led to marriage, and every time we are sore at each other—it happens in every marriage—we have a convenient scapegoat. We say it was the dogs' fault.

Although we had both been married before, neither of us had children. We both wanted one or two, and they came, and having Alice and then Phyllis has been a wonder and a joy. So we became a family, and there is no nicer word in the English language than "family," and no nicer feeling than being part of a loving family.

I realized I was pregnant for the first time while I was shooting a movie called *Weekend in Havana,* in 1941. Some people have said that I looked better in that movie than in any other, so maybe pregnancy agreed with me. Dorothy Manners, the Hollywood columnist, wrote at the time: "Pregnancy agrees with Alice Faye. She's never looked so beautiful. Her eyes have a new sparkle."

After Alice was born, I didn't accept any picture assignments for a year, so I could be with my brand-new baby exclusively. It was a marvelous year for me. When I returned to work, in *Hello, Frisco, Hello,* I was given the beautiful song "You'll Never Know," and I think that must have been my reward for being such a good mother. That song has been closely identified with me ever since.

I was pregnant again, with Phyllis, when I shot *The Gang's All Here* in 1943. So I worked through my two pregnancies and have always felt that working helped me through those lovely but trying periods.

The historians Will and Ariel Durant once called the family "the nucleus of civilization," and I buy that. The family is your anchor in a snug harbor. Wherever I am, whatever

I am doing, all I have to do is think of my family and I get that lovely, warm glow inside. I know that no matter what I might do, those people—husband, daughters, grandchildren—are there for me, and will always be on my side.

I grew up in that kind of family. My grandmother encouraged me with her love and prayers. My parents protected me, taught me, and loved me. My two big brothers were always there to help me fight my battles when I was young and assisted me in my career in later years.

I feel so sorry for those people who have never known what it is like to have the warm blanket of family love. But other, nonfamily people are a different story. I have had a few good friends in my lifetime, but when I stop to count, there haven't been that many I consider true friends. I remember reading once something Henry Adams wrote: "One friend in a lifetime is much; two are many; three are hardly possible."

I feel this way. If you have a handful of really good friends in your lifetime, you are one very lucky person. I have had that handful, and they have helped me enormously, and I value those friendships like pure gold.

There haven't been many really close, long-lasting friendships. One of the closest, longest-lasting has been with Betty Sharf. We were in the chorus together, back in my early days in New York. When I got into the movies I asked Betty to come with me and be my stand-in, and she was with me throughout my career. Walter Sharf was my musical director, and I introduced Betty to Walter. They have had a happy marriage and they are still great friends of mine. Two of my other closest, dearest friends have passed away—Florence and Clark Swanson. Clark was the frozen food king and both of them were wonderful people and very high-quality friends.

But, friends aside, I find many people are difficult to deal with and often impossible to get along with. Most people can make you downright miserable if you let them. One of my toughest battles is the one I fight in trying to tune people out. It isn't an easy thing to do.

People, I think, can be like food. Many of them are just too rich, too fattening to be good for you. They want things from you. They gossip too much. They have mean, nasty thoughts. They are jealous, envious, bitter.

I am very sensitive to what other people are thinking about me. I pick up those nasty vibes very easily. They may be smiling and sweet and pleasant on the surface, but I can tell that, deep down, they are full of resentment. I get hurt easily when I trust those surface sentiments and don't probe for what lies underneath. In my lifetime I have been hurt a lot. So I have to be very careful, and I am.

That, of course, explains why I am slow to make friends. I am, perhaps, too suspicious, too sensitive, too careful. It takes me a long time to warm up to people. I have dozens, maybe hundreds, of casual acquaintances, but only a very few people I consider close and dear friends. That way, I lessen the risk of getting hurt if a supposed friend knifes me in the back. (I forget who it was that said, "A true friend is someone who will knife you in the front." Maybe it was Phil who said it.)

I believe I have, over the years, developed a knack for judging people and a talent for weeding out the unscrupulous ones from the ones who might be OK. When a girl is young and people say she is beautiful, she gets a lot of men hanging around and has to develop that talent for pure self-protection. I did.

Now, when I meet someone new, I can generally size him or her up in short order. If I think that person wants something from me, my antennae go up and a message is flashed to my brain: "Watch out for this one, Alice, old girl. Caution! Beware!"

To a greater or lesser degree, all of us have that ability. There are many poor souls who are gullible and accept everyone at face value. But the majority of us have some sort of built-in mechanism that allows us to judge strangers. We are occasionally wrong in those snap judgments, but generally we are on the money.

But we must have some friends. They are an essential part of life, and we would be poorer without any friends at all.

There are some, I know, whose family relationships leave a lot to be desired. Those unfortunates have my sympathy. I have some acquaintances whose family ties have completely broken, snapped off like matchsticks. They have severed all ties with their children—or vice versa—and never see any of their relatives. They profess not to care. They say they are better off without them. They pooh-pooh such sentimental claptrap as birthdays and holiday gatherings. They are, I believe, whistling into the wind. I am sure that, when Christmas or Thanksgiving rolls around, they are desolate. Christmas particularly can be a miserable holiday for people who are alone.

So I suggest that, whatever caused the rift in your family, you mend it. Even if it wasn't your fault, swallow your pride, call your relations up, tell them you are sorry, visit them bearing gifts—make the effort to reestablish contact. As the years go by, you will find the need more and more to have family around. Maybe you can't stand your son-in-law or Uncle Jim Bob, but you don't have to live with them. No matter how boorish Uncle Jim Bob can be—and we all have somebody like that dangling from our family tree—he is family, and that means he is someone you can turn to if you need help. And somebody to ease your loneliness when you simply don't want to be totally alone anymore.

For many people the problem with family is the in-laws. You may adore your son, but your daughter-in-law is a horror. Or your spouse's mean old sister. Or your brother's wife. Or, that butt of so many jokes, your mother-in-law.

I was lucky, mother-in-law-wise. No problems there. Phil's father I never knew. He died soon after we met. So no problems there either.

I had many friends as a girl growing up in New York. And many more when I started dancing. But none of those friendships lasted too long. I envy people who have had friends for fifty or sixty years, childhood friends from the old neighborhood who are still friends in their young-elder years.

I think I might have had a lasting friend in Tyrone Power. (It is possible for a man and a woman to be friends without any romance being involved, you know.) He was a very wonderful person, kind and generous and giving. We were in three films together, and when you do a film together you are as close as two people can be. If there are flaws in someone's character, that's when you will discover them. But I never found any major flaw in Tyrone Power's character.

Henry King directed us in *In Old Chicago* and *Alexander's Ragtime Band*. (The other film we did together, *Rose of Washington Square,* was directed by Gregory Ratoff.) The big scene in *In Old Chicago* was, of course, the re-creation of the catastrophic Chicago fire. And King and the studio went all out to make that a spectacular sequence. I was not allowed on the set that day—no women were permitted. In those chivalrous days, women were protected—maybe over-protected, but it was a lovely thought. King felt that it would be too dangerous for us gals to be on the set during the fire, which was really a huge and potentially perilous blaze. So all the women you saw on the screen fleeing from the fire were actually stuntmen wearing women's clothing and wigs.

For reasons I no longer remember, King decided that Ty, Don Ameche, and I should take flying lessons. He was a pilot himself, and I guess he just felt we would enjoy sharing his passion for flying. So he enrolled us in a school, and we had to go out to the airport once a week—or maybe it was twice—

and take those lessons. Don and I dutifully took our lessons, and, although they were fun, I never caught the bug. But Ty Power did. He went on to solo and eventually got his pilot's license.

I remember Henry King tried to persuade me to keep on with my instructions. He said flying was such a marvelous experience. "I do some very constructive daydreaming when I'm flying," he said.

"If I am going to do any daydreaming," I said, "I'll do it with both feet on the ground."

That was the end of Alice Faye, aviatrix.

Having shared experiences like that is one basis for a lasting friendship. Common interests is another. If you find people with whom you have shared experiences and with whom you have a commonality of interest, cultivate them as friends.

Family is something else again. You can't choose your family (other than your husband or wife); they are thrust upon you, and you have to make the best of what you get.

People—whether they be family or friends—are all in-dividuals. Each has his or her quirks. And you have to accept them as they are, quirks and all, because that's the way they are. You can't change them, so don't bother to try.

There are all kinds of people, and maybe that's good. In my travels, and down through my busy life, I've met and gotten to know people of every size, shape, and sort.

Some people look like prunes, because that's the way they are—prunelike. They think like prunes and act like prunes. They don't like anybody or anything, and it shows on their faces, with their downturned mouths and their un-happy eyes. They have a lot of trouble digesting their food, so they keep popping Tums in their mouths all the time. They make very poor friends. Other people have sunshine in their eyes, smiles on their lips, and songs in their hearts. They eat well and sleep well and they make wonderful friends. Look for the sunny people, but try to avoid the prunes.

Of course, some of us seem to have a need to be around people who are difficult. Maybe these people have a touch of masochism in their souls, or something akin to that.

We are all different, and we all have our individual likes, dislikes, peculiarities, and habits. When you make a friend, or get married, or have a child—whenever you become closely associated with another person, no matter how it happens—you have to accept the bad with the good, the peculiar with the normal. The quirks are part of the works. They are the price you pay for having a relationship and, by and large, it is really a small price. It is a bargain. Most human idiosyncrasies are amusing rather than annoying and can easily be borne.

When I talk to people in my travels for Pfizer, I always get new evidence of the oddness that is part of the human condition. Listen to the voices of some typical Americans.

"I have terrible arthritis," one woman told me. "The only thing that seems to help me is sex. But I just can't seem to get my husband to cooperate."

"I've given up on people completely," another lady said. "I think people are no damn good. The only person who gives me any comfort is my parakeet."

"I play pool every afternoon from two until five," a young-elderly man said. "If it wasn't for my regular afternoon game of pool, I think I'd go off my rocker. But I have to be very careful who I play with, because Charley cheats."

"I can eat anything," a lady who was sitting next to me at a lunch said, "except chocolate-covered raisins. They give me terrible heartburn."

I remember a screenwriter once told me that a big, fat novel could be written about everybody who ever lived. I believe him. Each one of us is such a masterpiece of personality oddities and strange behavioral patterns that the main character in that novel would be almost beyond belief. Then superimpose on that the twists and turns of the average life, the joys and the tragedies, the laughs and the tears, and you have the stuff of a major work of fiction.

But it isn't fiction at all, it is reality.

I'm sure my own life could make a novel, and I'm trying to be very objective when I say that. Many best-selling works of fiction have been based on lives of less achievement than mine. The cold facts are that I started with virtually nothing and made it to the point where, in 1940, I was the number-one box office female star in America.

Phil's life may be even more remarkable than mine, in the sense that he is such a great character. I think I am reasonably normal—some quirks, of course, but mostly I am a straight arrow—whereas my dear husband is a mass of quirks.

Phil and Bing Crosby used to go hunting together a lot—in Baja California, in the High Sierras, in Colorado, and all over—and Phil would come back with these wonderful tales of the great meals he had prepared over a campfire out in the woods. He and Bing would bag a few quail or a string of trout, and Phil would turn them into a veritable feast with nothing but a few twigs and a frying pan. And I know he is a marvelous cook in the kitchen. But for some reason the outdoor barbecue stumps him.

But that's human nature. That's what makes Phil Phil, and it is things like that that make all of us the fallible creatures we are. Fallible but, by and large, lovable. Maybe it is the very fact of our fallibility that makes us lovable.

At any rate, we are all individuals. And we have to be accepted despite—or maybe because of—our individuality. Which brings me back to where I started this chapter. We all need the comfort and solace of having family and friends, or preferably both, around us.

In many families, I know, frictions develop. That is inevitable. There are hurt feelings. There are slights—some real, others imagined. Somebody says something that Aunt Minnie thinks is a reflection on Uncle Willie's character and so, for thirty-eight years, Aunt Minnie and Uncle Willie have not spoken to Aunt Dora and Uncle Gus. You can't invite both couples to the same family function or the fur will fly.

That's normal in most families, but it is nonsense. When all is said and done, the only people you really can count on are the members of your family. If you feel somebody said something that hurt you, talk it out with that somebody. Don't let some insignificant little bit of conversation rob you of the consolation of your family.

And the same thing applies to your friends. Good friends are so rare that you should fight to keep them. And truly good friends will talk to you, so if you think one of your pals has done something to you you don't like, or if you've heard he or she said something about you behind your back, talk to that friend and iron it out. Chances are it was all some sort of misunderstanding in the first place.

There is nothing worse than loneliness. And the only real defense against loneliness is having family and friends around you. If you cultivate those relationships in good times, they will be there to help you when times are bad.

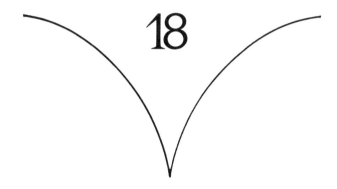

18

Throughout these pages you have probably noticed that I quite often used the term "young elders." I much prefer that to "senior citizens," which always sounds a little phony to me, or any of the other common names given to people who are sixty-five or beyond. To me, "young elders" conveys the concept I want to get across, which is that, although we may be getting on in years chronologically, we are—or at least we should be, and can be—still youthful in spirit and attitude.

But I want to stress here that, although my words are primarily directed to the young elders—after all, the title of this book implies that it is aimed at those who are Growing Older—what I have to say is also, I believe, valuable to younger readers. The earlier in life one begins to think about taking care of oneself, the better. There is no such thing as starting too soon to take care of your body. In fact, it is much easier for you if you do start when you are young.

It is hard for someone over sixty-five, who has never done much of anything about exercising, or watching his or her diet, or seeing a doctor, suddenly to begin doing all those good things. It is relatively easy for someone who is in his or her thirties or forties or even fifties to begin thinking in those terms. It may not be a cinch, but the younger you start, the cinchier it is. The longer you wait, the tougher.

I realize that many people in their early years, and even in their middle years, feel they are too busy to bother with such things. The rat race consumes all their time and energy. They are too busy trying to make a buck, trying to support a family, trying to have a little fun, to worry about tomorrow. And, furthermore, tomorrow, to young people, seems so far away that they don't concern themselves with it. But fortunately fitness has become fashionable. People are taking time to work out a little, to take care of their bodies, to consider their health. I think that is a marvelous thing, and I hope the trend continues.

There is, however, more to preparing for healthy and happy young-elder years than going to the gym twice a week for an hour. All the components of a healthy life for young elders that I have talked about in this book are equally important—exercising, watching what you eat, stopping smoking, staying active mentally, and seeing your doctor regularly and following his or her advice.

I believe that the ideal would be if people began a program containing all five of those suggestions as early in life as possible. Even in their childhood. (If you never start to smoke, then you don't have to go through the trauma of withdrawal.) So it is up to us, as parents and grandparents, to instill in our children and grandchildren those good values. It is something that can and should be done.

For example, that suggestion about seeing your doctor

regularly and following his or her advice. When our children are young, we take them to see a pediatrician regularly. We feel it is a necessity that they get a good, healthy start in life. Then, as they grow, we usually take them to see a doctor often—once a year, or more if there is any medical problem. However, that usually stops when they become teenagers. Why? Mostly because teens generally are bursting with good health; if you aren't healthy then, forget it. (The only doctor a teenager usually consults is a dermatologist, for acne.)

Because of our neglect, then, our children get out of the habit of seeing a physician regularly. It is not uncommon for a person not to see a doctor for ten or twenty years, from the time of the last childhood disease at, say, age twelve, until he or she gets a physical exam before marriage in the twenties.

Similarly, during those years the young person probably does little or no exercise, other than normal activity. And those are the junk food years, when a person gulps down breakfast (a cup of coffee and a piece of Danish pastry) in time to get to work on time, grabs a quick lunch at the nearest fast-food joint, bolts a frozen TV dinner in five minutes to get to the bowling alley on time. Young people go to bed late, get up early (except on weekends, when they often sleep around the clock). They probably smoke, they probably drink, they may even take drugs of one kind or another.

That, of course, is the life-style of the young and normal. It isn't a healthy life-style, and a lot of young people never make it to middle age because of those risky habits. But it is a product of our culture, for better or worse (mostly worse).

I urge you young elders to try to get your children and grandchildren to begin taking care of themselves right now. I know that they will probably say, "Oh, pooh," or words to that effect. They can't be bothered. They have too many other things on their minds. They don't have the time. They feel fine, so why rock and roll the boat?

But if you present them with some facts—and your local

health association will arm you with plenty of facts—about how they could very easily die unless they start taking better care of themselves, maybe you will get your point across. Also tell them that what you are suggesting won't take a lot of time, or money, and will be fun as well as beneficial. Maybe then you'll start to make an impression on their thick, stubborn young skulls. You might tell them that the world is changing, and some of the changes are good, but some of them are not so good. In fact, I think the world is, by and large, going to pot (and I am not trying to make a joke about drugs).

I am constantly appalled by what is happening in the world today. Consider the deplorable business of child abuse, child molestation, child stealing. When I was a kid, running loose on the streets of wicked New York, we were really very safe. I don't recall any instances of any of that, although I suppose there must have been some. But my mother and grandmother would let me play in the city streets, and I don't think they ever worried about my safety. Today, though, even in affluent and fancy suburbs, you cannot put a baby outside in a playpen to get a little sun. Who knows what creep could come along and steal the poor child, or worse? It has become a psychopathic world.

Young people today have a very difficult life. There is all the crime. There is the specter of drugs. There is the financial burden of today's society. There is the threat of nuclear war and nuclear catastrophe. There is the "greenhouse effect" and the depletion of the ozone layer and the polluted seas and acid rain and all the other products of our technology. I don't envy my grandchildren, because I think the problems their generation are bound to face will be almost too much.

Yet in other respects they are fortunate. If science keeps striding forward as rapidly as it has in the recent past, the future has great promise. There will probably be further advances in the treatment of cancer and heart disease and even

Alzheimer's disease. There may be new and better and safer methods of organ transplants. There will be advances in genetics that are exciting and a little frightening, too.

But despite all the progress, human nature will always remain the same, and this is the major problem. Unless people change their attitude, which is highly unlikely, nothing will really change. Unfortunately, we humans are basically greedy and grasping creatures. We may have moments of compassion and kindness, but they are fleeting. We have our men of genius, but many more men of narrow-mindedness and crassness. We are selfish, and because of that we really hurt each other much more than we help each other. We may go to church on Sunday, and talk piously about loving our neighbor, but it is all Sunday talk. On Monday, we go right back to knifing our neighbor in the back. There are exceptions, of course. Many of them. But I believe my assessment of the human animal is basically correct.

I think if we all took life a little easier, the world would be a better place. We should lighten up a bit. Take a few minutes to smell the roses. We rush too much, push too much, shove and elbow and try to be first in line, when being second is really no disgrace and no terrible tragedy. We are so concerned with being number one that we forget that the rest of the crowd has some rights, too. And, while we are pushing and shoving and elbowing, the parade is passing us by. We are so busy trying to protect our own selfish little interests that we miss the golden opportunity to see the marvelous things this world has to offer, to taste the joys of the good life, to smell those lovely roses.

I am doing a lot of philosophizing here, and I don't blame you if you say, "Who is she to preach to us?" You're right about that; I really have no right at all, when I can hardly get out of my own way. But I do have my ideas, and, since this is my book, I guess I can say what I want.

What is most important, however, is not my philosophy

of life, such as it is, but rather my thoughts on Growing Older but Staying Young. I got off on this tangent because I wanted to stress the fact that my ideas on this topic apply equally to both the young and the young elders, that you are never too young to start.

Encourage your children and grandchildren to begin taking care of themselves. And maybe they will be the ones to encourage you to do the same.

It is so easy to procrastinate. Life is full of ways to put things off until tomorrow. "I'll get around to it soon" is a favorite stall. Or "I'll start Monday." Or "When the weather is better" or "The next time I have a free hour" or any of those old wheezes. The point is that it is terribly easy to put things off, but terribly difficult to buckle down and get started. What I want you to do is say to yourself, right now, "This is something I have to do, for the sake of my pride and my personal satisfaction, and I am going to do it and I am going to start right this very minute."

It doesn't matter how young you are, or how old you are. It doesn't matter if you feel and look good, or feel and look rotten. The only thing that matters is that we can all feel and look better. We can all improve.

Begin today. Not tomorrow or next week or next payday. Begin today, this very moment.

How?

Start by standing up and taking a few deep breaths. There, you have begun. That wasn't so hard, was it? You might next do one of the standing exercises I describe in Chapter 7. And at your next meal, whether it be breakfast, lunch, or dinner, start limiting what you eat. Don't change your menu now—maybe you won't have to change your menu at all—but simply eat a bit less than you have been eating. And don't add butter to your bread (you'll find, after a few days, that you hardly miss it). And try drinking your coffee black and don't sugar your morning cereal and cut down on all sorts of fats and oils and salts and sugar. Cut down, but don't necessarily cut out entirely; if you cut way down, you will be doing enough for the moment. Then, maybe later, you can cut them out completely.

See? You are well on your way to Growing Older but Staying Young. And it has been easy.

That's one of the great things about the ideas I have advanced in this book, I believe. You can do it all so easily, without any major wrenching of your life-style, without any great expense, without any trauma to your body or your soul. You simply begin with a little exercise, a little care in what and how you eat. Then you make sure that your mind is as occupied as your body, and you check with your physician— and you are well on your way.

I know people who say, "Well, that's all well and good, but I am too set in my ways to do anything like that." That's a lot of poppycock. None of you is so set in his or her ways that you can't stand up for a few minutes and take some deep breaths, or can't change your eating habits to the extent that you eat a few bites less at each meal.

Admittedly, it can be difficult for someone who has been a smoker for many years to quit smoking. Difficult, but not impossible, because millions of people have done it. It may also be something of a problem for someone who is inactive to find something to do, some way of keeping active. But again, this is far from impossible.

Begin slowly. Begin by doing a few of the simple exercises, or by taking a walk for fifteen minutes or a half an hour. Begin by watching your diet a little more closely. Then move on to the other parts of the program. And soon you will find yourself feeling younger and looking younger.

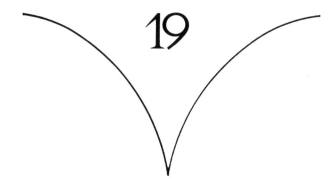

19

When I travel for Pfizer Pharmaceuticals and speak to groups of young elders, I usually talk for a few moments and then ask my audience if they have any questions for me. They almost always have a few, and generally the same questions are repeated wherever I go and whomever I speak to. Because of that, it occurred to me that you might be interested in some of the questions I am asked most frequently. If my audiences when I speak are curious about certain things, it stands to reason that my readers would have the same curiosity about the same subjects.

So here are the questions people seem to ask me most often (and, of course, my answers to those questions):

Q: What was it like to kiss Tyrone Power?

A: It is interesting how, after all these years, Ty Power still seems to retain his magic and his sex appeal. The ladies almost always open my question-and-answer session by asking me what it was like to kiss him, as I did throughout the three pictures in which we were costars, *In Old Chicago*, *Alexander's Ragtime Band*, and *Rose of Washington Square*. All I can say is that kissing Ty was a heavenly experience. We were always good friends—platonically—and the kissing was part of the job. But it made the job a very pleasant one.

Q: What was it like to kiss Don Ameche?

A: It's funny how people are so curious about Hollywood kissing scenes. I suppose the underlying question is always, Well, did that kiss lead to anything more? A screen kiss is not like a kiss on the porch swing or in the backseat of the car. It is part of acting, and as such it is first written into the script by the writer and then directed by the director. The writer usually has some stage directions as to how he wants the kiss to look, and the director has his own ideas. So before you get to kiss the guy, you are told how to pucker, where to look, what to do with your arms and hands, and on and on. In addition, there are dozens of technicians hovering over you—the makeup person rushing in to touch up your lips, the hairdresser with a final comb out, the lighting man with his meter against your cheek. When you finally kiss your leading man, it is all about as romantic as balancing your checkbook.

But, to answer the question, kissing Don Ameche was pleasant, too, because he was always a good friend. And I got to kiss a lot of other handsome men—John Payne, Robert Young, Spencer Tracy, Rudy Vallee, Dick Powell, Warner Baxter, and many, many more. Except for the occasional bad breath—if the kissing scene was after lunch and the leading man had had onions on his hamburger—it was always a nice way to make a living.

Q: What was it like to work with Shirley Temple?

A: Basically, it was awesome. I worked with Shirley in two films—*Poor Little Rich Girl* and *Stowaway*—and she was incredible. Her talent never stopped. She could be difficult, however. It wasn't temperament so much—her mother tried very hard not to spoil her, and to have her act normally—it was simply that she was a little child. And all little children have their bratty moments. If they get a little tired, they become whiny and petulant, and Shirley was a normal little girl, so she had her less than angelic moments, too.

Q: Is it true that you and Betty Grable didn't get along?

A: No, that is not true. As I said earlier in the book, that was something that the studio publicity department started, made up out of whole cloth to get people excited about seeing us in the movies we did together. In those days feuds were thought to make the public interested, so there was the Jack Benny–Fred Allen feud, the Walter Winchell–Ben Bernie feud, the Bette Davis–Constance Bennett feud, and several others. Betty and I actually got along very well, and I considered her a good friend up until she died. Studio publicity departments were notorious for inventing things about us actors that were absolutely untrue. One of my early studio biographies, for example, reported that I had studied opera and hoped to resume my studies and have a career in grand opera after I finished acting. Some people still believe that, but it was a complete fiction.

Q: What was your favorite picture?

A: No actor really has a favorite picture. Every picture I did has some pleasant memories for me. You naturally remember with particular fondness the pictures that were most successful, and for that reason I loved the ones I did with Tyrone Power and films such as *Little Old New York* and *Tin Pan Alley.* I also was very pleased with *Lillian Russell,* because it gave me my best dramatic part. And, of course, one always remembers one's first fondly, so *George White's Scandals* will always be near and dear to my heart. But you remember others for other reasons. As I mentioned earlier in this book, *Hollywood Cavalcade* was great fun because of the pie-throwing fight I had with Buster Keaton. Who wouldn't have enjoyed doing that?

Q: What was your least favorite picture?

A: Again, many films had moments—some had a lot of them—that weren't fun. And, of course, we tend to dislike the films that bombed, such as a bit of nothing I did called *Barricade.* But I could not single out any one as my least favorite, because even *Barricade,* although it was panned by the critics and people stayed away from the theaters where it was showing in droves, had been pleasant. There were some wonderful actors in the cast, and I got to sing a nice song—"There'll Be Other Nights"—even though it was cut out of the film before it was released.

Q: What song that you introduced did you like best?

A: I guess it would have to be "You'll Never Know" (from *Hello, Frisco, Hello*) because, in the first place, it has become a standard and it always makes a singer feel proud when a song he or she sang first goes on to become a standard. And, in the second place, "You'll Never Know" won the Oscar as best song in 1943, and that is another source of intense pride.

Q: Would you ever act again?

A: I would love to, under the right conditions and circumstances. I wouldn't want to do anything too demanding, but I would love to have a part on one of those nighttime soap operas like "Dynasty" or "Knots Landing" or "Dallas." Those shows have such huge casts that nobody works too hard; the work load is spread around among a dozen or more people. So if somebody made me an offer on a show like that, I'd do it. Or a nice part in a movie or a television miniseries. I'm available, but I'm not out looking for work.

Q: What do you think of today's movies?

A: I think there are some good ones and some bad ones, as there have always been. I know it is cozy to think back to the movies of the '30s and '40s and remember how marvelous they were, but don't forget when we do that we are remembering the great ones. For every marvelous movie we made back then, the studios poured out a dozen Grade B or lower stiffs. We tend to forget the bad things and remember only the good. There were plenty of bad movies made back then, as there are today. The difference is that a lot of the bad movies made today are considered Grade A.

Q: Which one of today's leading men would you have liked to have acted with?

A: Being a normal girl, I think it would have been jolly good fun to work with Paul Newman and Robert Redford. Some of the other fellows—De Niro, Pacino, and that crowd—seem a little too intense for my taste.

Q: Do you watch much television?

A: I watch quite a bit, but I am not a slave to it. There are some programs I enjoy, but, having been a singer and dancer originally, I miss the variety shows. I used to enjoy being on them myself, and I enjoyed watching them, too. I hope that they will make a comeback, although I doubt it. They have been replaced by videos and the MTV channels on cable TV and all that. I watch some good sitcoms and good dramatic shows and the news, and when Phil and I are together he usually has on a baseball or football or basketball game, so I watch those, too.

Q: What's the secret of your long marriage?

A: I believe I've answered that in this book, but, for the record, I think it's a combination of several factors—luck has a lot to do with it, and the fact that Phil and I are not always together and we give each other lots of space, and the fact that we both had previous marriages that failed so we wanted this one to work, and the fact that we both wanted a home and family life—all those things helped. It is also very nice that we happen to love each other a lot.

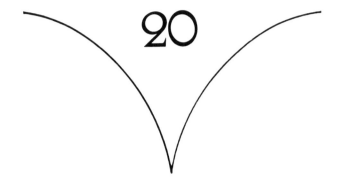

20

Nowadays I go out on the road, spreading the good word about health on behalf of Pfizer Pharmaceuticals, ten or twelve times a year. It is always fun for me—not the traveling, as I have told you, because I don't like that, but the chance to meet and talk with people. But, fun or not, these trips are almost always occasions for some wild and crazy happenings. I thought you might like to hear about some of the adventures of Alice Faye, Girl Traveler.

This is traveling made as easy as possible, because the good and kind folks at Pfizer always meet me, wherever I am supposed to go, and escort me to my hotel. I have gotten to know the Pfizer representatives around the nation that way, and without exception they are a fine group of young men and women.

What is nice is that wherever I go, to a big city or a small town, the people know me and remember me and seem to feel warmth toward me. Once, after I had spoken to a large group of young elders in San Diego, a man came over to me and, without a word or any encouragement on my part, he proceeded to give me a big hug and a kiss. Now I like a kiss and hug as well as the next person (of course that depends on who the next person is), but I do think it is more friendly if I know the kisser and hugger. And I didn't recognize this gentleman.

"Hey, Alice!" he said. "You were great."

"Why, thank you very much." But I could see he expected more. He stood there, looking at me as though I should say something else.

"Don't tell me you don't remember me," the man said. Oh, so we are going to play guessing games, I thought to myself. I hate people who call you on the phone and don't give their names, and expect you to guess their identities. This was a variation on that game, and I wasn't going to play.

"No," I said. "I'm very sorry, but I don't remember you. Should I?"

"Well, it's been about forty years," he said, "but back then we were pretty close."

"Forty years! Has it been that long?" Now I was stalling, because if he said we were close, then I should remember him. And I usually have a pretty good memory.

"Give or take a year, yeah. I'll give you a hint—radio."

Then suddenly it all flashed into my head. This man had been the producer of the radio show Phil and I did back then—and it *was* about forty years ago. Once I placed him, everything shot back into my mind, and he and I had a grand reunion, talking about those good old days.

I prefer appearing in small- to medium-sized halls. My favorite places to appear are at conventions, where Pfizer sets up a booth and I can just mingle with the people as they walk by. To actually make a speech, as I sometimes am called on to do, is hard for me. But I do it, because it is my job.

When I meet people individually, things are much easier for me. I thoroughly enjoy it when a person comes up to me and just starts chatting away. Usually, people ask some of the questions I mentioned in the previous chapter. Sometimes I can tell that they want to ask about Phil and me, but they are slightly hesitant—they don't want to embarrass me if we have been divorced and they don't want to sadden me if he is dead. So they sort of beat around the bush, and I can sense it, and I try to put them at their ease by saying, "Oh, I'm still Mrs. Phil Harris, and the old boy is still alive and kicking."

Once in a while some people are under the impression that I have scientific credentials. I guess it is because of my association with Pfizer. They see me standing there, in front of all the scientific displays, and jump to the assumption that I am some sort of advanced scientist.

One of them once called me "Dr. Faye." "Dr. Faye," this eager lady said, "what do you think of the current research into cellular and molecular hyperdivision in middle-aged white rats?" (Or something like that.)

I quickly set her straight. "I am not a doctor," I said. "Not even a nurse. I am just a movie actress who knows who to go to to ask questions, and you should ask that gentleman over there"—and I pointed to one of the Pfizer reps—"about your white rats."

I've had people come up to me and tell me about the pain in their right side, and ask me if I thought that meant the beginnings of an ulcer, and I've had them ask me what I recommend for persistent headaches, for allergies, for arthritis, for everything under the sun. I always point them in the direction of the nearest Pfizer man or woman, and smile at them and sign my autograph and they go away happy. Usually, Dr. Michael Freedman, who is director of geriatric medicine at the New York University Medical Center, travels with me, and he fields those medical and scientific questions.

The most embarrassing thing that ever happened to me, however, was really not my fault. I was in Pittsburgh. The Pfizer people, as usual, met me at the airport and took me to my hotel. I went up to my room to get freshened up. They told me I should go down to the Paradise Room (I forget the actual name of the room they said, but it could have been Paradise), where there was a meeting of some group and I was scheduled to make a little talk.

So, on schedule, I went down to the lobby, asked where the Paradise Room was, and went into it. A large group of people were milling around, and I began circulating. "Hello, I'm Alice Faye," I said. And they were always very pleasant. "How lovely to see you," they would say. "I remember you in *Rose of Washington Square.* You look terrific!" They seemed like a very nice group of people. I didn't see my friends from Pfizer anywhere, but there were a lot of people, so I might have just missed them.

I went up to where there was a head table and a microphone, and I asked a man who seemed to be in charge when I should give my little talk. "Right now would be fine," he said. And he clinked on a glass and everybody quieted down. "Folks," he said. "We have a treat for you. You all remember Alice Faye from all those great movies. Well, she is right here, and she is going to talk to you." And I got a very nice round of applause.

I made my little talk about the Pfizer Five—the five elements that go into good health: Exercise. Eat right. Don't smoke. Stay active. See your doctor regularly. (All the main points I have covered in this book.) They seemed to be very attentive, a good audience.

Just when I was winding up, I saw one of the Pfizer people at the door waving at me. I waved back and kept on talking.

When I finished, I got another very nice round of applause. And the man in charge got up to speak. "Thank you very much, Miss Faye," he said. "That was a very interesting talk. On behalf of all the members of the Pennsylvania Society of Nuclear Physicists, I want to express my appreciation."

I had gotten into the wrong room! We all—me and the nuclear physicists—had a good laugh once we had sorted that one out.

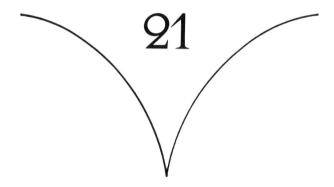

21

Many years ago, at some forgotten point in my early career, I happened to meet a man who was one of the world's great pitchmen. He was one of those people who can sell anything to anybody—iceboxes to Eskimos and room heaters to Africans. I forgot what he was selling when we met—snake oil, or something like it. Anyhow, we got talking, and I asked him what was the secret of his selling success.

"Little lady," he said, "selling something is simple. All you have to do is tell 'em what you're going to tell 'em, then you tell 'em, and then you tell 'em what you told 'em."

Well, I skipped the first part of his formula in this book. I didn't tell you what I was going to tell you. I just jumped in and started telling you what I wanted to tell you. But now I think it would be a good idea to tell you what I told you, to recapitulate and wrap it all up in a few pages.

There are, I believe, five things you must do if you are to Grow Older but Stay Young.

1. You have to exercise, keep your body moving, keep the muscles flexible, keep the heart pumping and the blood circulating and everything working as smoothly as possible.

2. You have to watch what you eat. And by that I mean primarily a balanced diet and not too much food. Push the plate away before you are overstuffed.

3. Try not to smoke. And don't drink to excess. And, of course, take no drugs of any kind—other than what your doctor prescribes.

4. Keep yourself busy and keep yourself active. That is exercise for your mind. You just can't sit around and watch the daisies grow, or you'll be pushing them up.

5. See your doctor regularly, but, equally important, do what he or she tells you to do. Get your prescriptions filled, and take your medicine as the doctor suggests.

Those are the five essentials for people who want to continue to be youthful looking and youthful feeling.

I also told you about some ideas I have about makeup, about hairstyling, about what to wear and what not to wear. But those are really only gilding the lily. First, you have to have a lily worth the gilt, and the five points I just reviewed are the way to preserve and protect your body and your spirit.

The whole point of this book is that none of us has to grow old badly. That phrase "grow old gracefully" is something that's within our power to achieve. Obviously, some of us are going to show more signs of age more noticeably and more quickly than others. That's just the luck of the draw. But even those who show the signs early—people who go prematurely gray, for example—can look young. Mostly it is a matter of how you *feel* inside. If you feel young and full of energy, you will look younger. And to feel young and full of energy, you have to, first, be in the best possible health you can be, and, second, have the best possible attitude you can have.

That's where Growing Older but Staying Young comes in. If you follow my five points—when I go out and speak on behalf of Pfizer Pharmaceuticals, I call them the "Pfizer Five"—then your chances of feeling your best and looking your best are considerably improved.

So exercise, eat right, try not to smoke, keep busy and active, and see your doctor regularly and do exactly what he or she tells you to do. Then you will be ready for whatever the years throw at you, and you will grow old gracefully.

And, by the way, it helps if you have a sense of humor, too.